THE WISDOM OF MILTON H. ERICKSON
Human Behavior and Psychotherapy

Ronald A. Havens

IRVINGTON PUBLISHERS, INC.
NEW YORK

Irvington Publishers, Inc.,
Executive offices: 740 Broadway, New York, New York 10003
Customer service and warehouse in care of: Integrated Distribution Services, 195 McGregor St, Manchester, NH 03102, (603) 669-5933

The Wisdom of Milton H. Erickson: Human Behavior and Psychotherapy was originally published as Sections I and II of *The Wisdom of Milton H. Erickson* (New York: Irvington Publishers, Inc., 1985).

Cover photo courtesy of Elizabeth Erickson:
Milton H. Erickson under his favorite tree.

Library of Congress Cataloging-in-Publication Data

Erickson, Milton H.
The wisdom of Milton H. Erickson.

Reprint. Originally published: New York, N.Y.:
Irvington Publishers, c 1985.
    Contents: 1. Hypnosis and hypnotherapy—2. Human behavior and psychotherapy.
    1. Hypnotism—Therapeutic use. 2. Psychotherapy.
I. Havens, Ronald A. II. Title.
RC495.E74 1989   616.89'162   88-31440
ISBN 0-8290-2413-1 (v. 1) Formerly ISBN 1-55778-155-9
ISBN 0-8290-2414-X (v. 2) Formerly ISBN 1-55778-219-9

1 3 5 7 9 10 8 6 4 2
Printed in the United States of America

TABLE OF CONTENTS

PREFACE TO THE
PAPERBACK
EDITION

Milton H. Erickson, M.D., is most widely recognized for his innovative contributions to the fields of hypnosis and hypnotherapy. This hardly is surprising given that virtually all of his professional publications and lectures centered upon these topics. Scattered throughout his journal articles and presentations, however, are numerous comments reflecting his basic underlying views about human functioning and psychotherapy. When these insightful but frequently overlooked comments are separated out and organized into a meaningful gestalt, as I have attempted to do in the present volume, a powerful new perspective on these issues emerges. In fact, the quotations presented in the following pages seem to represent the foundation for a revolution in our approach to the entire therapeutic enterprise.

There is a companion to the present volume which provides a separate compendium of Erickson's observations about hypnosis and hypnotherapy. Although it is not absolutely necessary to become familiar with his views on hypnosis and hypnotherapy in order to comprehend his views on people and psychotherapy, it is highly recommended. Hypnosis was a focal context for the development of much of the wisdom contained in the present book and, thus, a familiarity with Erickson's approach to hypnosis may clarify further his comments about psychotherapy and human nature.

I hope that you will find Erickson's words as revealing and useful as they have proven to be for me. As you read through these pages, however, please keep in mind that this is merely a synopsis of his views. I am quite sure that there was more to Erickson than we will ever know.

ACKNOWLEDGEMENT

Many thanks are due to my friend and colleague, Dr. Richard Dimond, for his encouragement and contributory ideas and for his assistance in copying many of the quotations eventually used in this book. Thanks also to Sandy McGuire and Maryanna McCall for their patience and skill in typing from the original handwritten manuscript which was a genuine nightmare of inserts, corrections, and bibliographic details. My wife, Marie, deserves special mention and thanks for her warmth, sacrifice, support, and editorial review of my work.

Finally, the author wishes to acknowledge the following journals, publishers, and individuals who generously provided permission to use quotations from sources copyrighted by them:

American Medical Association (*Archives of Neurology and Psychiatry*), American Psychiatric Association (*American Journal of Psychiatry*), American Psychological Association

(*Journal of Abnormal and Social Psychology and Journal of Experimental Psychology*), American Society of Clinical Hypnosis (*American Journal of Clinical Hypnosis*), American Society of Psychosomatic Dentistry and Medicine (*Journal of the American Society of Psychosomatic Dentistry and Medicine*), British Psychological Society (*British Journal of Medical Psychology*), Brunner/Mazel, Elsevier Publishing Co. (*Psychosomatic Medicine*), Encyclopaedia Britannica, *Family Process*, Grune & Stratton, Jay Haley, Harper & Row Publishers, Irvington Publishers, Journal Press (*Journal of General Psychology* and *Journal of Genetic Psychology*), Herbert S. Lustig, M.D., Macmillan Company, Merck, Sharp & Dohme (*Trends in Psychiatry*), Physicians Postgraduate Press (*Diseases of the Nervous System*), Psychoanalytic Quarterly Inc., Plenum Publishing Corporation (for Appleton-Century-Crofts), Science & Behavior Books (for Meta Publications), Society for Clinical and Experimental Hypnosis (*Journal of Clinical and Experimental Hypnosis*), Springer Verlag New York, W. B. Saunders (*Medical Clinics of North America*), William Alanson White Psychiatric Foundation (*Psychiatry*), Jeffrey K. Zeig, Ph.D.

In accordance with the procedures requested or required by the relevant parties, acknowledgement is hereby provided that portions of the copyrighted material specified below have been reprinted by permission of the copyright holders:

Abridged sections from "Basic Psychological Problems in Hypnotic Research" by Milton H. Erickson, M.D. in *HYPNOSIS: Current Problems*, edited by G. H. Estabrooks. Copyright © 1962 by George H. Estabrooks. Reprinted by permission of Harper & Row Publishers, Inc.

Bandler, Richard & John Grinder. *Patterns of the Hypnotic Techniques of Milton H. Erickson, M.D.* Volume I, Science & Behavior Books, Inc. Palo Alto, California, copyright © 1975 by Meta Publications.

Erickson, M.H. Development of apparent unconsciousness during hypnotic reliving of a traumatic experience. *Archives of Neurology and Psychiatry*, 1973, *38*, 1282–1288, Copyright © 1937 by American Medical Association.

Erickson, M.H. Negation or reversal of legal testimony. *Archives of Neurology and Psychiatry*, 1938, *40*, 549–555. Copyright © 1938 by American Medical Association.

Erickson, M.H. Demonstration of mental mechanisms by hypnosis. *Archives of Neurology and Psychiatry*, 1939, *42*, 367–370, Copyright © 1939, American Medical Association.

Erickson, M.H. Hypnotic investigation of psychosomatic phenomema: Psychosomatic interrelationships studies by experimental hypnosis. *Psychosomatic Medicine*, 1943, *5*, 51–58, Copyright © 1943 by the American Psychosomatic Society, Inc.

Erickson, M.H. The therapy of a psychosomatic headache. *Journal of Clinical and Experimental Hypnosis*, October, 1953, 2–6, Copyright © by The Society for Clinical and Experimental Hypnosis, October, 1953.

Erickson, M.H. A clinical note on indirect hypnotic therapy. *Journal of Clinical and Experimental Hypnosis*, July, 1954, 171–174. Copyright © by The Society of Clinical and Experimental Hypnosis, July 1954.

PREFACE

The material in this book was compiled in an attempt to clarify the concepts and attitudes necessary for an effective application of the Ericksonian forms of therapy and hypnosis. It is not a compilation of Ericksonian techniques nor is it a theoretical analysis of Dr. Erickson's work. It is, instead, simply a collection of the observations and ideas that Dr. Erickson himself presented in numerous publications and lectures in an effort to communicate the wisdom that guided his interventions. It is an effort to capture and to convey the essential ingredients of his solution to the most fundamental problem facing us all, i.e., how to enjoy and use life to its fullest and how to enable those around us to do the same. Some people spend more time than others grappling with this problem and many, such as psychotherapists, earn their living doing so. Ultimately, however, this issue forms a common denominator between us all in our universal search for insights, understandings, and truths about ourselves.

Rarely in this search are we presented with straightforward observations about how people operate or about what factors influence human behavior. Information about people typically is so tightly embedded within a specific theoretical framework that it is impossible to determine fact from fancy. As we read various texts on personality theory, hypnosis, and psychotherapy, we are confronted by the contradictory theoretical assumptions of either the Freudians, the Jungians, the Adlerians, the Rogerians, the Skinnerians, or some other prominent school of thought. Each of these theoretical systems views people in an entirely different light and each leads to entirely different dogmatic observations and recommendations about what to do and when. As a result, human nature and human behavior continue to be confusing mysteries for most psychotherapists; a phenomenon we participate in without real understanding and attempt to influence in ourselves and others without much effect.

It would be especially significant, therefore, if someone came along who had taken the time and effort simply to observe what people actually do and what variables actually influence their behavior. It would be even more significant if this person had translated these observations and had demonstrated how to apply them for the benefit of oneself and others. Anyone could certainly benefit from such accumulated wisdom.

Milton H. Erickson did just that! He observed, he noticed every detail, and he applied his observations in his practice of hypnotherapy. He devoted his life to careful observation of himself and others and, as a result, he became more familiar with the nature of people than perhaps anyone else before or since. As a consequence, he learned how to enable others to utilize potentials they did not know they had and he helped them resolve personal and interpersonal problems that no other professional had been able to touch.

And he tried to teach others the wisdom he had accumulated by those years of observation. He wrote and he lectured and he taught throughout his entire professional career. He taught, in fact, until several days before his death on March 25, 1980 at the age of 78.

This book is a distilled synopsis of what this remarkable man observed and what he taught throughout his lifetime. Naturally, the wisdom contained in these pages should be of tremendous value for anyone seriously interested in becoming an effective hypnotist or psychotherapist. Erickson was a master of both and his comments on these endeavors may represent the best advice and instruction available.

On the other hand, his general knowledge about people represents such a unique perspective of such proven value that it deserves serious consideration even by social scientists who believe that both hypnosis and psychotherapy are useless or irrelevant to their interests. Every psychologist, sociologist, anthropologist, or other professional involved in the study of people should find it worthwhile to learn what Erickson had to say because his observations have significant implications for an understanding of all aspects of human functioning.

What Erickson noticed about people provides a perspective on ourselves which seems to be descriptively accurate, objectively valid, conceptually challenging, and totally beyond the boundaries of any existing paradigmatic perspective. Here, at last, is a person who told us simply what people are and what they do without imposing a set of biased and limiting assumptions or theoretical constraints between his perceptions and the world around him. All theoreticians, researchers, and clinicians owe it to themselves to take a fresh look at people through Erickson's perspective. What they see may or may not strike them as useful, but it is guaranteed to give them something to wonder about and it is likely to open their awareness to aspects of human behavior that they had previously ignored.

A similar comment could be made about people interested in becoming more aware and more effective, no matter what their age, vocation, role, or status. Erickson's wisdom is universal in its application and impact and, as such, it deserves to be deciphered and shared with everyone. The basic perspective Erickson taught in the lecture hall was identical to what he taught to his patients in his office. In both instances he was simply attempting to teach others a way of being and perceiving that would motivate and enable them to use their inherent capacities and previous learnings to cope most effectively with the realistic demands of their lives. It is hoped that this book will facilitate that process in some small way for students of psychology and psychiatry, for practitioners of therapy, counseling, and hypnosis and even for nonprofessionals interested in learning about themselves and others.

AN INTRODUCTION TO MILTON H. ERICKSON, M.D.

Milton H. Erickson was probably the most creative, dynamic, and effective hypnotherapist the world has ever seen. Not only could he hypnotize the most difficult and resistant patients imaginable, he could even do so without their conscious awareness that they were being or had been hypnotized. He hypnotized people by talking about tomato plants in a certain way, by describing the objects in his office in a certain way, and even by shaking hands in a certain way. There were, in fact, several colleagues who refused to shake hands with him after he had successfully demonstrated his handshake induction upon them. During a lecture in Mexico City in 1959 he hypnotized a nurse in front of a large audience using only pantomime gestures, a feat made even more impressive by the fact that this Spanish-speaking nurse had no idea when she volunteered that she was to be a subject in a demonstration of hypnosis. In a sense, the variety and effectiveness of

Erickson's hypnotic inductions defies imagination, though none seems less likely to be effective than his "Shut up, sit in that chair there and go into a deep trance!", an induction technique that he made work.

As a psychotherapist he was equally creative and effective. It is doubtful that many therapists would conclude that effective intervention should involve teaching patients how to squirt water between their teeth, stepping on patient's feet, sending them out to climb mountains, having them strip naked in the office and point to each part of their bodies, or having them eat a ham sandwich. Yet these are some of the strange strategies that Erickson employed with outstanding success, and with each patient he seemed to generate another unique and almost outlandish intervention. His psychotherapy style was so completely innovative and his success rate was so high that many of his patients were people referred to him by other psychotherapists or were those other psychotherapists themselves.

It should come as no surprise, therefore, that Milton H. Erickson has been described by other hypnotherapists in some of the most laudatory terms imaginable. At various times he has been referred to as a master hypnotist, as a psychotherapeutic wizard, and as the world's foremost authority on hypnotherapy and brief strategic psychotherapy. In 1976 he became the first recipient of the only award presented by the International Society of Hypnosis: the Benjamin Franklin Gold Medal. This medal was inscribed *"To Milton H. Erickson, M.D. — innovator, outstanding clinician, and distinguished investigator whose ideas have not only helped create the modern view of hypnosis but have profoundly influenced the practice of all psychotherapy throughout the world."*

In December of 1980 several thousand professionals descended upon Phoenix, Arizona to pay posthumous tribute to him and to participate in workshops and presentations on his hypnotherapeutic techniques. This *International Congress of Ericksonian Approaches to Hypnosis and Psychotherapy* had been preceded for years by a constant stream of professionals to training sessions in his office in Phoenix. Elsewhere throughout the country and throughout the world workshops on Ericksonian techniques have become almost mandatory inclusions in the programs of professional conferences in psychotherapy and hypnosis. Books by and about him have become bestsellers almost overnight and Dr. Ernest L. Rossi has even edited a four-volume collection of almost all of his numerous published and unpublished articles. In short, it probably would not be an exaggeration to state that Erickson has had a greater impact upon the human services professions than any other single individual since Freud.

It is somewhat ironic that the peak of his public recognition should have occurred only after he reached the age of seventy. Prior to that time the value of his work was acknowledged only by a relatively small group of devoted followers. His therapeutic techniques were rarely mentioned in textbooks on psychotherapy and even books and articles on hypnosis by some of the most prominent scientific investigators in the field often gave no more than a brief mention of his techniques or research contributions. In fact, it is easy to get the impression that Erickson was intentionally ignored by many of his contemporaries. Whether or not this was the case, the fact remains that he was a maverick to a large extent, a unique person with strong and unusual convictions, and an unselfconscious person who was not afraid of confrontations. His background and professional activities both explain and demonstrate this quite clearly.

Erickson was born on December 5, 1901, in the now defunct town of Aurum, Nevada. His pioneer parents eventually moved "east" in a covered wagon and settled on a farm in a rural section of Wisconsin. Even as a child he experienced the world in ways that were quite different from those of his friends and relatives. Aside from an intense curiosity and a general reluctance simply to accept the beliefs and superstitions of his rural community, Erickson's world was different from others for physiological reasons as well. For example, he had an unusual form of color blindness that enabled him to perceive and enjoy the color purple but little else. As a result, he surrounded himself with this color in later life and eventually became quite interested in the hypnotic induction of color blindness. He was also arrhythmic and tone deaf, phenomena that led to his intense interest in the effects of alterations in breathing patterns associated with the "yelling" that others called singing. In addition, he experienced dyslexia. The various difficulties created by that anomaly actually intensified his familiarity with and interest in the meanings and implications of words. It is especially intriguing that a person who would eventually become one of the world's experts on the use of language did not learn to talk until the age of four and even then, because of his arrhythmia and tone deafness, spoke in a rhythm totally unlike most Americans. Various experts have compared his speech pattern to that of a Central African tribe, that of a Brazilian tribe, and that of a Peruvian tribe.

Finally, Erickson experienced a lifetime of physical ailments beginning with a life threatening bout of polio at age 17 and culminating in a second case of polio in 1952. Although he was able to recover almost completely from the total paralysis of his first bout with polio, the unusual second case took a more severe toll. For most of his later years he was confined to a wheelchair with no real use of his legs, little or no use of his right arm, and restricted use of his left arm. Eventually, he was able to use only half of his diaphragm to speak and his mouth had become partially paralyzed as well. In addition he suffered from chronic intense pain which he moderated with autohypnosis.

In spite of his many physical discomforts and handicaps he remained active and therapeutically effective until his death on March 25, 1980. Throughout his lifetime he was forced to overcome an incredible variety of adversities, but he had a way of turning all of his difficulties into advantages and valuable opportunities for learning. He was fond of saying that life's difficulties were merely necessary roughage. Few other people have ever made more effective use of so much roughage.

Perhaps because he was so atypical physiologically, Erickson began observing and influencing the behavior of others while still a small child. For example, he enjoyed walking to school early through the new fallen snow, leaving behind him a crooked path. His journey home that afternoon was then made more interesting by observing how many other children had walked to school following his crooked path instead of creating a straighter one of their own. Similarly, as he slowly recovered from the total paralysis of polio he spent many days simply observing the behavior of those around him and gradually, as a result, he became remarkably sensitive to body language and developed methods to elicit needed help from others without asking for it directly.

He used his skills at influencing the behavior of others during a one-man canoe trip of over 1200 miles that he undertook as physical therapy in the summer of 1921 following his first year as an undergraduate. When he began this summer trip he was so weak from the aftereffects of polio that he could swim only a few yards at a time and could not even lift his canoe out of the water. He had some beans, some rice, and slightly more than two dollars with him to purchase additional supplies. Yet without ever directly asking for assistance he managed to elicit enough fish from curious fishermen, money from odd jobs along the river, and help in getting his canoe over dams to manage quite well. In fact, by the time he returned to Wisconsin he could swim a mile, could carry his own canoe, and was more than ready to begin his second year of classes at the University of Wisconsin.

During the first semester of his sophomore year at the University of Wisconsin, Erickson experienced one of his many spontaneous autohypnotic phenomena. This experience seems to have had a profound effect upon his thinking and may have set the stage for his subsequent introduction to hypnosis by Clark Hull. Erickson had decided that he wanted to earn some extra money by writing editorials for the local newspaper and he had planned to write them by using an ability he had discovered when he was younger. This ability consisted simply of sometimes being able to dream the correct solutions to arithmetic problems. Accordingly, he planned to study until 10:30 P.M. at which time he would go to bed and awaken at 1:00 A.M. to write the editorial he hoped he would have created in his dreams in the meantime. He awoke the next morning with no memory of having written the editorial, yet there it was, carefully placed under his typewriter. He decided not to read that editorial or any of the others he produced in the same mysterious manner and submitted to the newspaper that week, but each day he looked in the paper to see if he could find one he thought he might have written. He discovered that he was unable to recognize his own editorials, each of which had been published, and concluded that "there was a lot more in my head than I realized." That experience also led him to conclude that he should begin to trust his own understandings and not allow them to be distorted "by somebody else's imperfect knowledge."

In spite of these and other similar experiences, Erickson did not begin to think in terms of hypnosis until the end of his sophomore year when he observed a demonstration of hypnosis by Clark L. Hull. Erickson was so excited by this demonstration that he subsequently managed to get Hull's subject to allow Erickson to hypnotize him and he spent the following summer hypnotizing anyone who would cooperate with him.

He reported on the various experiences and conclusions accumulated over that summer during a graduate seminar on hypnosis conducted by Clark Hull the following fall. Erickson's conclusions conflicted sharply with those of Hull, who approached hypnosis from an experimentalist and learning theorist point of view. Hull's emphasis upon a standardized approach and de-emphasis of the importance of any inner processes of the subject were directly contrary to Erickson's own observations and this difference of opinion led to considerable acrimony and estrangement between the two men. According to Erickson, Hull regarded his views as "unappreciative disloyalty and willfull oversight" (Erickson, 1967). Erickson, in turn, has since labeled Hull's standardized approach an "absurd" and "futile" endeavor that disregards "...the subject as a person, putting him on a par with inanimate laboratory apparatus..." (Erickson, 1952).

Needless to say, Erickson was unable to convince Hull that he was wrong. Instead, Hull formalized his views further, conducted a series of experiments based upon them and published this material in his book, *Hypnosis and Suggestibility: An Experimental Approach*, in 1933. The conceptual and experimental assumptions underlying this landmark book formed the foundation for the modern scientific view of hypnosis, a view that continues to reject or to conflict with Erickson's perspectives.

Hull was also unable to convince Erickson that Erickson was wrong. Undaunted by Hull's rejection of his perspective, Erickson continued to utilize and to do research in hypnosis. He consulted with others at the university including Dr.

William Blackwen of the Psychiatric Department and Dr. Hans Rees, a professor of neurology, regarding the design of a research project to determine the inherent or basic differences between hypnotized and non-hypnotized subjects. This and other research projects on hypnosis were begun and conducted on an extracurricular basis throughout the remainder of his academic career. Thus, by the time he had completed his B.A. in 1927 and his M.A. in psychology and M.D. degrees in 1928 at the University of Wisconsin, he had developed an extensive background and high level of expertise in this area.

Along the way, he found it necessary to solicit the help of a psychiatrist-lawyer to prevent his dismissal from graduate school for dealing with the black art of hypnosis. When he began his internship at the Colorado General Hospital (1928-1929) he emphatically was forbidden even to mention the topic of hypnosis under the threat of dismissal and refusal of his state licensing application. Characteristically, however, Erickson was able to continue his work in hypnosis by associating with the Colorado State Psychopathic Hospital where he eventually received a special residency in psychiatry following his internship and licensure.

During the year following his special residency in psychiatry (1929-1930) he was an Assistant Physician at the Rhode Island State Hospital for Mental Diseases after which he joined the Research Service of Worcester State Hospital in Massachusetts. When he left, four years later, he had become chief psychiatrist on the Research Service.

From 1934 to 1939, he was Director of Psychiatric Research at the Eloise Hospital and Infirmary in Eloise, Michigan where he subsequently was promoted to Director of Research and Psychiatric Training, a position he held until 1949. While in Michigan, Erickson was a prolific writer and researcher in the field of hypnosis. The productivity of this period is even more remarkable given his joint appointment in psychiatry at Wayne University College of Medicine from 1938 to 1948 and his joint appointment as a professor in the Graduate School of Wayne State University from 1943 to 1948. He also was a Visiting Professor of Clinical Psychology at Michigan State University in East Lansing, Michigan for a brief time.

Erickson met his second wife, Elizabeth, while teaching at Wayne State University where she was a psychology student and graduate assistant. His first marriage had ended in divorce and when he married Elizabeth in 1936 he brought three children with him from that marriage. Subsequently they had five additional children, which may partially explain why Erickson was so familiar with and referred so often to the process of human development and early learning in his lectures.

In 1948, primarily for health reasons, the Ericksons moved to Phoenix, Arizona where, after working briefly in a local institution, Erickson established a private practice. The remainder of his life was spent in Phoenix where he continued to practice in an unpretentious office at his home. Eventually, his cramped office became cluttered with various mementos and presents from patients who had flown from as far away as New York or Mexico City to be treated by him. In his later years he would meet with eight or more people at a time in his small office to teach and to conduct hypnotherapy. These people came to Phoenix to learn from the master, though a number of them reportedly ended up learning more about themselves and less about hypnotherapy *per se* than they had originally expected.

Erickson himself was unconcerned that his cramped and cluttered office did not accurately reflect his growing stature and prestige in the field. In fact, his first office had held only a card table and two chairs, but he had defended his decor by stating "*I* was there." He may have been unpretentious but he was not unconvinced of his own prowess and competency! As quoted in Zeig (1980), Erickson states, "As for my dignity ... the hell with my dignity. (Laughs) I will get along all right in this world. I don't have to be dignified, professional." He also says, "And I am very confident. I look confident. I act confident. I speak in a confident way ..." These two comments are a remarkable summary of Erickson's life and style and provide some insight into the man who was so convinced that he was right and so unconcerned with what others thought of him that he was able to challenge the traditional assumptions and techniques of the scientific and professional community and to blaze his own unique path.

During the early 1950's Erickson undertook a series of teaching seminars in hypnosis throughout the United States and other countries. As a result of his presentations before a group of professionals in Chicago, the Seminars on Hypnosis Foundation was established. Many of the members of this teaching group, of which Erickson was the senior member, had participated in his early seminars in Chicago. Subsequently, the Seminars on Hypnosis Foundation evolved into the American Society of Clinical Hypnosis — Education and Research Foundation.

In 1957 Erickson became the founding president of the American Society of Clinical Hypnosis. This society provided a more clinically oriented alternative to the previously formed Society for Clinical and Experimental Hypnosis. SCEH had been established in 1949 within a Hullian scientific tradition and it had maintained that experimental tradition quite emphatically. As a determined opponent of the theories and hypnotic techniques of this tradition and as a dedicated clinician, Erickson founded ASCH and served as its president from 1957 to 1959. In 1958 he became founding editor of the *American Journal of Clinical Hypnosis* and served in this capacity until 1968, during which time he was able to provide a forum for authors whose interests and theoretical assumptions may not have been appropriate for SCEH's *Journal of Clinical and Experimental Psychology*.

From 1967 on, Erickson received an increasing amount of recognition for his psychotherapeutic skills in addition to his hypnotic abilities. Although his publications during that period continued to focus upon the techniques and considerations underlying hypnosis, various books about him began to appear that focused instead upon his therapeutic interventions (cf. Bandler & Grinder, 1975; Haley, 1967; 1973). These publications brought him to the attention of a much broader audience and ensured an ever-increasing following.

Prior to his death Erickson had received numerous honors and awards. He was a Life Fellow of the American Psychiatric Association, the American Psychological Association, and the American Association for the Advancement of Science. He had received a diplomate from the American Board of Psychiatry and had been a member of the American Psychopathological Association. The July, 1977 issue of the *American Journal of Clinical Hypnosis* was dedicated solely to his work in honor of his 75th birthday. The list of achievements and honors could go on, but the point simply is that Milton H. Erickson was a person worthy of our careful study and attention; a unique, effective, and influential hypnotherapist who evidently knew something very special about people and translated that knowledge into effective hypnotic and therapeutic strategies.

HOW AND WHY
THIS BOOK WAS
CREATED

Unfortunately, Erickson never translated his unique body of knowledge and learning into an organized, detailed account of his conceptual framework. Although he was a prolific author (over 140 scholarly articles and co-author of several books) and lecturer, he rarely provided more than brief, general glimpses of his underlying system of thought. Erickson once stated, "If I started teaching by precision I'd bore them." (Zeig, 1980) and it is safe to say that his audiences were rarely bored. As a result, however, there is no single publication of his that offers the interested and motivated reader a genuine or complete sense of the wisdom that guided him throughout his hypnotherapeutic career. The observations and conceptual perspective underlying his strategies have remained remarkably elusive and it seems safe to assert that there are few hypnotists or therapists in the world who could rightly claim to understand Erickson's approaches thoroughly or to be able to utilize them as effectively and creatively as he did.

As a consequence of the conceptual void left by his reluctance to do more than hint at the underlying observations or concepts that guided his work, Erickson's traditionally trained colleagues often tended to view his interventions as illogical, confusing, mysterious, magical, irrelevant, or even irreverant. Apparently it was easier for many to dismiss him as a show-off, a charlatan, or a lunatic than to undergo the perspective shift and careful observation necessary to appreciate what he had to offer.

On the other hand, even among his followers there often seemed to be much confusion as to whether his effectiveness should be attributed to him as a person, to his unique perspective and wisdom, or to the specific techniques he developed and described. Those who held fast to the first view formed little more than a cult following and the third view was held primarily by those who had become particularly effective at imitating his physical and verbal mannerisms and in training others to do likewise.

Although it is obvious that Erickson was a powerful personality and that imitation of his mannerisms may be effective under some circumstances, it also seems apparent that only by learning the fundamental concepts and information that guided him, and thus adopting his underlying perspective, can we hope to understand the logic of his actions or to create similar interventions on our own. Erickson may not have presented a direct or complete explanation of his work, but fortunately he did attempt to communicate bits and pieces of it to others. Comments pregnant with meaning and implications are scattered throughout his lectures, case histories, and research summaries like the parts of a complex jigsaw puzzle.

Unfortunately, the actual meaning and implication of each of these jigsaw statements are apparent only within the context of the entire pattern of his knowledge. Each of his general comments seems to be meaningful alone, but that meaning shifts and changes slightly as other statements of his are read or heard. The problem with understanding what Erickson was trying to tell us is that each of his comments is almost invariably interpreted within our own framework of understanding because his was so unique and, thus, difficult to comprehend. The meaning we tend to impose upon his comments is not necessarily the meaning he intended to communicate and, paradoxically, it is probably impossible to comprehend the meaning he was trying to communicate until we can comprehend it *in toto* from within the framework of his specific perspective.

The limitations generated by this natural distorting and misunderstanding process were very familiar to Erickson. He typically admonished his students in the following manner: "So, I warn all of you, don't ever when you are listening to a patient, think you understand the patient, because you're listening with your ears and thinking with your vocabulary. The patient's vocabulary is something entirely different." (Zeig, 1980, p. 58). Later on he adds the comment that "We always translate the other person's language into our own language." (Zeig, 1980, p. 64). Even Dr. Ernest Rossi, who spent many years studying with Erickson, was subject to this error for which he received the following admonition: "You were placing *your* meaning on my words. But what was *my* meaning?" (Erickson & Rossi, 1981, p. 211). This may be the ultimate question facing all students or practitioners interested in becoming proficient in an Ericksonian approach or anyone interested in learning what this man knew about people. What was *his* meaning?

The idiosyncratic meanings of Erickson's conceptual comments and their presentation in a diversity of sources are major obstacles to a widespread appreciation and utilization of his wisdom. Furthermore, the amount of time involved in a thorough review and reorganization of his work to isolate and organize his more pertinent comments regarding the nature of people, the purpose of psychotherapy, etc. is not available to everyone who might be interested in doing so. By a lucky coincidence, however, my fascination with the work of Erickson and the granting of a sabbatical leave from my teaching responsibilities at Sangamon State University provided me with both the motivation and the opportunity to conduct such a review.

I began this project solely to satisfy my own personal need to understand once and for all what this incredible clinician had to offer. I had a purely selfish and admittedly grandiose desire to comprehend what Erickson knew, a desire that had not been satisfied by the numerous analyses of his work which I had read previously or by my relatively unorganized and cursory exposure to his numerous articles and books. Whenever I began to feel that I understood what he was saying, I would run into another quotation that confused me, added some new twist, or directly contradicted my original notions. Finally my patience ran out and I decided to use the time available to me to read everything of his that I could get my hands on and to consolidate in an organized fashion all of his comments that seemed to be direct expressions of his accumulated knowledge and basic observations. In essence, I hoped to create a concordance of Erickson's concepts and knowledge that would guide and direct my own thoughts, observations, and clinical activities.

The initial stage of this project consisted of a thorough and careful reading of Erickson's published works. At first it was necessary to rely upon the bibliography of his writings compiled by Gravitz and Gravitz (1977) to find these materials. However, the publication of his collected works by Rossi

(Erickson, 1980) facilitated this process considerably. Additional books, transcripts, and audio tapes contributed further insights and notable quotations. Eventually it was possible to review almost every publication by or about him prior to 1981.

As these books, transcripts, and articles were read, statements that expressed his general observations, basic concepts or underlying assumptions in any way were carefully noted. Such statements were rarely lengthy and usually were scattered rather widely through his writings, inductions, and speeches. In addition, I eventually decided to use only comments that were directly attributable to Erickson himself, a decision that eliminated much of the material in most co-authored works. Accordingly, what began as several thousand pages eventually was reduced to several thousand "significant" quotations of varying length and complexity.

Each isolated quotation was assigned to a general category on the basis of its predominant content. Those dealing with hypnosis were placed in one category, those dealing with therapy were placed in another, and those providing broad generalizations about people were placed in the third. All quotations in each category were reviewed and subdivided further into smaller groups in accordance with their primary topics. Eventually, all comments about the conscious mind were in the same file, all of those about the unconscious in another, etc.

Next, all of the quotations from each subcategory were spread around several large tables and small clusters of highly related or similar statements were created. It was quite startling to realize how frequently Erickson had discussed the same points over the years. Apparently he had referred over and over again to a fairly limited number of issues, sometimes repeating previous statements almost verbatim, typically adding new details or insights. It was somewhat comforting to learn that he had not undergone any dramatic changes in his perspective during his professional career. It simplified my task and seemed to emphasize the significance of his position.

As the statements assigned to each cluster were reviewed and organized, it became apparent that the material contained an inherent organization. In spite of their original separation in time, the statements within each category almost had to be organized in a specific hierarchical arrangement if they were to be understood. Some comments simply could not be appreciated until others were read. Similarly, there seemed to be a necessary hierarchy of importance to many of the topics covered. An understanding of what was conveyed in some categories seemed to form the foundation for what was said in others.

It is difficult to convey the impact created by my first thoughtful reading of the resultant condensed and organized collection of Erickson's words. What had emerged from my efforts was more than I could have anticipated or had any reason to expect. As I read through those organized quotations, an entirely new conceptual reality began to take form before me. When I had finished, the clarity, coherence, implications and seemingly unchallengeable validity of what I had read was overwhelming. Throughout the years Erickson had developed a view of reality, of people, of hypnosis, and of therapy that was simple, direct, and yet remarkably insightful. The how and why of his effectiveness as a hypnotist and psychotherapist suddenly became blatantly obvious and had an immediate effect upon me. As the scattered shards of wisdom organized themselves into meaningful gestalts, the truth and beauty of the final form became genuinely compelling.

Other readers may not experience the same opening up of new worlds of observation and understanding or feel the same impact upon their personal and interpersonal patterns of thought and interaction as I did. They may not even find anything new in these collections of quotations. After all, everything in them has been said before by Erickson and much of it has been summarized effectively or alluded to by others in their reviews of his work. At least for me, however, once the actual words of this man had been allowed to organize themselves in a fashion that enabled them to speak their whole message at once, they seemed to speak with a clarity and a directness that I had been unable to experience when reading them separately or as interpreted by someone else. Because of this, I quickly concluded that I had a responsibility to share what I had discovered in order to provide Erickson with a final forum before *his* words faded into the background and those of his well-meaning followers and interpreters began to replace them. The result is this book.

My first impulse was to publish only the set of organized quotations thereby providing readers with nothing more or less than Erickson in his pure form. However, it soon became apparent that this would be inadequate. A context needed to be provided for some sections, connections needed to be established between others, and the entire collection required an ongoing process of introduction and summary. I have not endeavored to present a theoretical analysis of Erickson's work nor to relate his work to other theories or research. I have merely attempted to facilitate the reader's comprehension of the material quoted.

An effort has been made to eliminate irrelevancies and to organize the quotations in such a manner that each section holds together as a coherent whole and does not read as a jumbled array of disconnected comments. No doubt there are instances where the original or intended meaning has been distorted by the decision to place a statement in a particular context. Every effort was made to avoid this and I believe that any instance where this occurs is rare and relatively inconsequential. In the interests of space, clarity, and the avoidance of undue repetition, not all of the quotations originally isolated and placed in each category have been presented here. As mentioned earlier, Erickson reiterated most of his fundamental points on a number of different occasions, and only those comments which capture the essence of his perspective most effectively were incorporated into this final product.

This is not a book to be read quickly and effortlessly. Every quotation requires careful consideration and integration with previous comments. Erickson knew what he was talking about. I hope I have succeeded in allowing his words to speak to you.

HUMAN BEHAVIOR

HUMAN
BEHAVIOR

The material contained in this section is the essence of Milton Erickson's success. All of his hypnotic techniques and psychotherapeutic strategies were derived from a perspective or approach to life that led to careful objective observations and understandings of people. Although an understanding of his perspective will not turn anyone into a master hypnotist or therapist, it should provide the framework or foundation and motivation necessary to learn how to be one. More importantly, perhaps, it may provide an attitude toward oneself and others that can generate a clarity of vision, a sense of purpose, and a philosophy of life that is genuinely liberating and that can initiate a new focus for the conduct of one's life and work.

CHAPTER ONE

OBJECTIVE OBSERVATION YIELDS WISDOM

Erickson maintained one fundamental orientation toward life that will be emphasized numerous times in this book. This orientation may have grown out of his heroic battles with life-threatening and crippling effects of polio as a teenager or, as I strongly suspect, may have emerged much earlier as an expression of his family's pioneer spirit. Whatever its time of origin or source, it runs as a connecting thread throughout his work, emerging over and over again in various contexts in one form or another. It provided his definition of normal versus pathological functioning, specified his goal of hypnotherapy, and guided the style of his hypnotherapeutic work. The significance of this fundamental orientation to life within the context of the present chapter, however, is that it generated his awareness of the necessity for careful, objective observation as opposed to theoretical constructs.

Erickson's fundamental orientation toward life, perhaps the central theme of his work, was that people must learn to recognize, to accept, and to utilize what actually is in order to meet their needs, accomplish their goals, and satisfy their purposes. Rather than lamenting, distorting, or denying the unpleasant facts of life or fantasizing about an easier, more ideal reality, Erickson proposed that people must experience and acknowledge the realities of their situation and apply whatever capacities they have in order to cope as effectively or purposefully as possible with those realities. He recognized that this often is a difficult or confusing task, but argued that to do otherwise is to create artificial restrictions, unnecessary handicaps, and unrealistic perspectives.

Erickson entered the fields of psychology, psychotherapy, and hypnosis with this orientation and applied it unerringly in those fields. As a consequence, he rapidly concluded that no single theory could explain or describe adequately the incredible variety and unique complexity of individual functioning. From his perspective, the use of theoretical constructs and generalizations about people was a lazy and inadequate method of describing individuals and a useless exercise in fantasy, as well. Accordingly, he did not subscribe to any particular theoretical perspective nor did he develop one of his own. Those who would search for the theory underlying his strategies are doomed to frustration and failure and those who would impose a theoretical model upon his techniques merely demonstrate that they have missed his major point altogether. The fact is that he did not have a theory of human behavior to guide him nor did he use a theory to develop his intervention strategies.

Erickson may not have used a theory to guide his interventions, but what he did during his therapy sessions was neither arbitrary nor magic. He often spent hours considering the structure and content of his interventions and rarely, if ever, relied upon intuitive hunches or trial and error, even though these sometimes seem to be the easiest explanations for his sometimes bizarre, always unique, strategies. Somehow, without depending upon a carefully constructed theoretical model of human behavior, Erickson was able to decipher the complexities of people and to elicit curative responses from his patients. The question is, of course, what secret wisdom or knowledge did he use to plan and accomplish these therapeutic breakthroughs.

Erickson's secret was an incredibly simple and yet audaciously revolutionary concept. He developed his remarkable understandings of how people behave purely by observing them very, very closely, open-mindedly, and almost naively. He did not sit in his office reading or thinking about how people operate — he watched them. He did not become immersed in theories which he then tried to apply to various patients — he noticed what his patients did and modified his thinking in response. Erickson's spectacular success was based upon his willingness to let people teach him what was real or true about themselves and not upon unique theoretical constructs. The marvelousness of his concepts is that they are descriptively accurate truisms about people and not mere speculations about imaginary dynamics. He learned how to intervene in and how to influence human thought and behavior in the same way that most people learn how to ride a bicycle as children. He paid close attention, he experimented, and he made notes of what happened. As a result, he had no more use for theoretical constructs than a child has for the notions of momentum or velocity when learning to ride a bike.

But Erickson observed in a manner and with an intensity not typical of most people. First of all, he observed himself in incredible detail internally and externally. Secondly, he observed others with an intensity that surpassed even the most self-conscious analysis. Finally, he unashamedly observed people other than patients. Almost everyone was fair game to satisfy his curiosity and to fill in the gaps in his understanding. He hypnotized his sisters and told them to undress in preparation for a complete physical examination just to see what they would do (they refused). Similarly, he attempted to induce other subjects to play practical jokes on their friends, to destroy prized possessions, to lie, to verbally abuse others, and even to steal. All of these "experiments" were carried out under carefully controlled conditions, but they indicate the lengths to which he was willing to go to obtain information. Even strangers in train stations and airports or members of his audiences became opportunities to note how people responded under various circumstances and in response to various stimuli.

Erickson's emphasis upon careful observation pervaded his teachings and lectures. Over and over again he emphasized the necessity of observing subjects with an open-mindedness and precision that most people can only approximate. It may seem odd to us that simply looking at what people do under various circumstances gave this man such a unique understanding of others that he became one of the most effective hypnotists and psychotherapists of all time and developed one of the most innovative and powerful conceptions of human behavior of the century. But, as Erickson often demonstrated, most of us are so *unobservant* that we would be lucky to notice a car careening toward us in broad daylight. As an example Erickson mentions the case of a woman wearing sandals who walked into his office with her husband (Zeig, 1980). Erickson noticed that the second and third toes of both feet of the woman were partially webbed, but both the husband and *the woman herself* were ignorant of that simple fact. On another occasion (ASCH, 1980) he described an incident wherein he had instructed a group of interns to observe silently an elderly woman lying under the covers in a hospital bed until they noticed something unusual that would suggest a diagnosis to them. After three hours of supposedly careful observation, none of them had taken notice of the seemingly obvious fact that both of her legs had been amputated in mid-thigh.

As mentioned in the brief biographical sketch in the beginning of this book, Erickson suffered from a series of perceptual and physical defects. It is apparent that his childhood dyslexia, tone deafness, arrhythmia, color blindness and his eventual bouts with polio caused him to pay closer attention than others do both as a form of compensation and because he did not automatically perceive or respond in the same way as others. For this reason, Erickson had a life-long ability to observe the details of human behavior and to notice things that others missed. This childhood ability eventually became a professional pastime or obsession that resulted in a general description and utilization of human functioning *par excellence*.

Before we move on to a review of his general observations regarding the nature of human consciousness, however, it may be informative and useful to examine briefly the details of the observations upon which these more general conclusions were based or from which they were derived.

Observations Regarding the Influence of Breathing Patterns

Possibly the clearest examples of perceptual deficits that led Erickson to notice things that most of us miss were his tone deafness and arrhythmia. As a result of these "deficiencies" Erickson became puzzled and curious in grade school about the behavior of his classmates and sisters whenever they listened to music or singing (cf. Erickson, 1980, Vol. 1, Chapter 16). For some inexplicable reason they began to move their hands and feet and bodies in regular patterns whenever music was played and what confused him most was that their breathing patterns all shifted in unison when one song ended and another began, even though none was actually singing ("yelling" to Erickson) at the time. Erickson felt no urge to move about in this manner and was unaware of any shift in his own breathing pattern. But he became intensely aware that his classmates consistently began humming the songs sung by soloists after awhile. Thus, what is commonplace, expected, and generally ignored by most of us became a source of considerable concern and interest to him because he did not naturally respond in the same way.

After some experimentation he found that when he mimicked the pattern of breathing associated with a particular song, those around him would begin humming or even singing that song and assume it was a tune that had just come to them out of the blue. (His questions about this phenomenon were met with rebuffs and disapproval, a response he later indicated merely stimulated his interest and observations further.)

Erickson's observations eventually revealed to him that a particular pattern of breathing could initiate not only humming or singing but even yawns, a discovery that he employed surreptitiously to interrupt recitations by classmates, to initiate yawning in an entire classroom, or even to disrupt the lecture of a boring professor. Eventually he became convinced that breathing patterns could be used to communicate a variety of messages in an unobtrusive and unrecognized fashion, a recognition that he often employed when inducing a hypnotic trance.

It is worth noting that young children were able to notice the intentional shifts in his breathing pattern and the effects of these changes even when adults could not. One two and one-half year old told Erickson that "you breathe me to sweep" and other children observed that he just breathes differently to get someone to go to sleep or to wake up. This and other demonstrations of the relative perceptiveness of children eventually had a profound influence upon his general descriptions and understandings of adult behavior, as will become apparent later.

Observations Regarding Learning About One's Body

When Erickson went through the process of re-learning how to move following the total paralysis created by his first bout with polio, he naturally was forced to pay close attention to a learning process most of us have long since forgotten. What he observed in himself he also noticed later in his children as they developed. These various observations eventually coalesced into an understanding of the essential characteristics or basic pattern of human functioning. Aspects of human development that most of us take for granted, rarely consider, or even ignore totally became of central concern for him at that time and what he observed eventually was incorporated into his basic model of human behavior and into his hypnotherapeutic strategies.

Location of Body Parts: One of the first things Erickson had to re-learn as he recovered from polio was how to locate and recognize the signals from the various parts of his body. His nurse would touch his hand or his toes or his face and he would try to guess where the sensation had originated. It took him a long time simply to recognize what each sensation meant in terms of location and intensity of pressure.

The difficulty of reconstructing an understanding of one's body parts, the relationship between them, and the location of stimuli from them gave Erickson a profound sympathy for the immense amount of learning confronting a developing child. He carefully watched his children go through this learning process and noticed the manner in which they gradually discovered their physical identity. He noticed their puzzlement when they first tried to grasp their right hand *with* their right hand, something that children apparently do before they learn that the object *is* their right hand. Then he watched them discover and explore their right hand with their left hand and vice versa. He observed the details of their examination of the location, movement and sensation of each finger, of each arm and of each leg. He noticed how they determined the location of one ear by feeling it with one hand and then with the other. All parts, he concluded, had to be located in relationship to all others.

Later he noticed that children became awkward and confused as they grow because the relative distances between these various body parts changes. The head gets smaller relative to the rest of the body and the arms and legs move farther and farther away from their original anchor points. New patterns of response in relationship to oneself and the environment have to be learned continuously. Suddenly, one day it is no longer possible to walk under the kitchen table; the child has grown too tall.

He watched children learn these and many other things about their bodies and about the relationship of their bodies to the world around them and he became increasingly aware of how many things people learn, know, and use every day but do not remember learning and do not know that they know. His appreciation for this aspect of human functioning eventually formed a cornerstone for his approach to hypnosis and therapy, but there were many other events and observations that led to, reinforced, and added to this insight.

Learning to Walk: Few people have paid more attention to the learning necessary for normal walking than Erickson. As he began to re-learn how to stand and how to walk (an endeavor he undertook in spite of the pronouncement of doctors that he would never again be able to walk) he watched and imitated his baby sister who was busy learning the same thing. In later life he still could describe in minute detail each step in the process, from pulling oneself up, to keeping the feet apart, legs uncrossed, knees straight and hips locked. He was aware of the remarkable range of adjustments necessary to maintain balance as the position of hands, head, or arms is shifted. He could analyze the variety of movements and sensations associated with moving one foot forward and then the other. And having learned to walk again he was able to look around him and say "You all can walk, yet you really don't know the movements or the processes." (Zeig, 1980)

Once again he was confronted by the incredible amount that people know but don't know that they know, by the incredible range of learning that everyone has in their background but seldom recognizes. His infirmities led him to look carefully at what the rest of us tend to take for granted (and thus ignore) and he was mightily impressed by what he saw. In a sense he seemed to be staggered by how little attention people give or need to give to their own behaviors, to their accumulated body of learnings, to their own potentials. People walk, dress, eat, talk, write, sing, and conduct the routine business of their lives without giving it a thought. And yet, as Erickson struggled to understand and re-learn all of these activities he became awed by them and by the richness of learning and the remarkable range of potentials they represented.

Observations Regarding the Meaning of Words

Whether in spite of or because of his failure to begin talking until the age of four, language held a particular fascination for Erickson as a child. He had literally read the unabridged dictionary from front to back by the end of the third grade, a feat that earned him the nickname, "Dictionary." For some reason, however, it never occurred to him that the dictionary was arranged in alphabetical order to facilitate the process of finding words in it. Whenever he wanted to find a word he began at the beginning and looked through every page until he found the word he was looking for. This time-consuming process did not bother him because he enjoyed reading the dictionary and finding out about words. Not until his sophomore year of high school did the purpose of the alphabetical structure occur to him, an insight accompanied by a blinding flash of light and followed by a somewhat sheepish reluctance to admit to his belated recognition of so obvious a fact.

Nonetheless, his ignorance of the structure of the dictionary enhanced his awareness of the meanings, implications, and nature of words. He loved word games, puns, metaphors, and the inherent flexibility of language. At times he would entertain himself by talking to a group of his classmates in terms that he knew would lead one to believe that he was talking about kites, another to believe he was discussing baseball, etc. The multiple implications of words literally fascinated him. For example, he was impressed that the word "run" can have at least 142 different meanings depending upon how it is used and that the word "no" uttered alone can mean at least 16 different things depending upon the voice quality, body language, and inflection employed.

This knowledge of the different meanings and effects of words enabled him not only to say different things to different people at one time, but also to say many things to a single person at one time. He employed his awareness of the multiple implications of words to communicate things that the listener was unaware of on a conscious level. More importantly, he also used it to understand what others were saying unconsciously. It may very well be that his familiarity with the multiple meanings of words allowed him to understand what others were saying in ways that neither they nor other listeners could hear or comprehend. Words were, to him, so flexible in meaning that he tended not to impose his own meaning upon them but rather listened for the specific, perhaps idiosyncratic, unconscious meanings that they had for the speaker.

Observations Regarding Nonverbal Communication

Erickson's awareness of the unconscious levels of communication going on constantly between people was further refined and enhanced by the effects of polio. While still almost totally paralyzed, his interactions with those around him naturally were highly restricted. As a consequence, he was pushed into a role of passive observer of the interactions of others. Once again what he saw and heard became a source of amazement for him because he noticed that the verbal and nonverbal communications between any two people frequently blatantly contradicted one another. Verbal agreement, for example, might be accompanied by a whole range of facial expressions, hand movements, body movements, eye movements, and even voice inflections that implied disagreement. Furthermore, he noticed that such messages of disagreement did not go entirely unnoticed, but often led to an "intuitive" sense that the speaker had not meant what the literal message had conveyed. The reality of this bi-level pattern of communication, perception, and response was overwhelming as he observed his family and friends interacting. This, in turn, added to his awareness that people constantly emit and respond to signals or cues of which they are totally ignorant or unaware.

Observations Regarding Physiological and Behavioral Patterns

Erickson's ability to "read" people, to know things that they did not know about themselves or to see through their attempts to hide information are legendary. When he joined the staff at Worcester State Hospital, the Clinical Director took him aside and advised him to "walk around with a blank face, your eyes open, your ears open." He could not have given this advice to a more receptive, responsive, or astute subject. Erickson immediately began refining his ability to decipher the meaning or implications of minor changes in physiological and behavioral patterns of functioning by writing down his observations about specific people. Later he compared his observations about a person and tried to find out what had occurred in the meantime that might account for any differences. Eventually, he had perfected his observational skills to such an extent that he could tell by a woman's walk or the way she sat in a chair whether she was having an affair; he could listen to his secretary typing and determine whether she had begun menstruating that day; he could determine that a woman was pregnant before she had any idea that she might be and on one occasion (Zeig, 1980) he described in remarkable detail the pattern of minute physiological changes associated with the onset of an active sex life.

In many respects Erickson was a master detective first and a master therapist and hypnotist only as a consequence. He noticed everything about almost everyone he met and he became proficient at organizing clues into meaningful patterns and deciphering their implications. No theory, no catalog of human behavior could possibly convey to an aspiring hypnotherapist the complexity and enormity of information available to Erickson as a result of his lifetime of careful observation. Each movement, each word, each inflection, each physiological characteristic of a person was observed, noted, and interpreted on the basis of his experientially acquired understandings. This book will attempt to convey his general understandings, but it will remain the reader's responsibility to use those understandings to acquire the kind of details Erickson himself found it difficult to convey.

Observations Regarding Cultural Differences

Erickson was thoroughly familiar with the cultural modes and mores of many diverse groups and recommended that all psychotherapists study cultural anthropology both as a way of gaining insights into the behavior of patients from specific cultural backgrounds and as a means of broadening their appreciation for the potential variety of human thought and behavior. Although he acquired a great deal of his familiarity with the idiosyncracies of diverse groups and nationalities by reading books, he first noticed the impact of various cultural beliefs and attitudes at an early age.

By the age of ten, for example, he had recognized how rigid and unmodifiable were his grandfather's traditional attitudes about planting potatoes. Even after young Erickson had planted a successful potato patch during the "wrong" phase of the moon and with the "eyes" pointed every which way, his grandfather remained unwavering in his original belief that there was a specific phase of the moon during which potatoes should be planted and that they should always be planted with the eyes pointing upwards. He found a similar rigidity in a neighbor who developed headaches whenever Erickson tried to explain the importance of crop rotation to him. During his sophomore year in college he had the opportunity to observe closely the unusual beliefs and behaviors of an ethnic farming community where the males were expected to (and did) develop headaches the day after sexual intercourse, where married men vomited their breakfasts, and where many aspects of life were governed by similarly atypical patterns of thought and expectation. Erickson was selling books in this rural community and, as such, he ate and slept with a different family each day. He took advantage of this opportunity to observe the intimate details of their lives and did not hesitate to ask questions in an attempt to understand the patterns of thought that led to the unusual events he observed.

In later years Erickson continued to expand his comprehension of the impact of imposed cultural values by studying the do's and don'ts of many different nationalities, ethnic groups, and even regions of the United States. His friendships with Margaret Mead and Gregory Bateson may have contributed to this interest, and his extensive travels on his teaching seminars necessarily exposed him to many diverse groups.

Erickson's interest in cultural differences provided him with more than just an awareness of the conceptual rigidities and learned patterns of response people inherit from their cultural traditions. It also enabled him to perceive psychopathological behavior in a unique light and to derive a unique understanding from those perceptions. For example, while on the Research Service of Worcester State Hospital he interviewed a catatonic schizophrenic who manifested a variety of bizarre behaviors and beliefs which struck Erickson as familiar. Eventually he was able to relate them to those of several primitive tribes, a discovery which puzzled him greatly because the patient obviously was quite unfamiliar with the beliefs and rituals of any of these tribes. These and other observations of the spontaneous development of identical patterns of thought and behavior among separate individuals throughout the world and throughout history led him to conclude that basic human thinking and emotion are very much the same from person to person in spite of individual and regional idiosyncracies. In other words, he observed that the human mind has an incredibly wide but finite range of potential patterns available to it and that everyone has the capacity to function within any one of those patterns. *The particular patterns that any given individual adopts or manifests, he realized, are a result of limitations imposed upon this original pool of potentials by culture and by the individual's unique experiential history.* He determined that given the right circumstances, any individual can and will produce the patterns typical of any disordered state and perhaps of any other individual or culture as well. He also realized that every individual has the capacity to adopt the perspective of others and the ability to adopt new, more useful perspectives under the right circumstances.

Relevant Quotations

The following quotations from various articles and lectures by Milton Erickson are presented to convey his emphasis upon the importance of observation in the development of scientific understanding and in the formation of clinical skills. Examples of his observational capabilities are also included.

It should be noted that many of the quotations used in this and the following chapters were taken from *The Collected Papers of Milton H. Erickson on Hypnosis* (4 volumes), edited by Ernest L. Rossi, published by Irvington Publishers in 1980. Where this is the case, the original date of authorship or publication has been placed in brackets at the end of the quotation in order to provide an orientation regarding the actual dates and sources of the various comments. A complete listing of the original references for this material can be found in the References section.

For the most part our knowledge of psychological processes has been achieved through clinical observations. [1937]

(In Erickson, 1980, Vol. III, chap. 16, p. 145)

Any discussion of hypnotic psychotherapy or hypnotherapy requires an explication of certain general considerations derived directly from clinical observation. [1948]

(In Erickson, 1980, Vol. IV, chap. 4, p. 36)

It is satisfying personally to offer theories and hypotheses, but it would be so much better to investigate actual phenomena. Research should be centered around phenomena, not around achieving fame by placing in the literature a well-argued theory intended to "explain" some unexamined manifestation. [1962]

(In Erickson, 1980, Vol. II, chap. 33, pp. 344-345)

In brief, we need to look upon research in hypnosis not in terms of what we can think and devise and hypothesize, but in terms of what we can, by actual observation and notation, discover about the unique, varying, and fascinating kind of behavior that we can recognize as a state of awareness that can be directed and utilized in accord with inherent but unknown laws. [1962]

(In Erickson, 1980, Vol. II, chap. 33, p. 350)

When I wanted to know something, I wanted it undistorted by somebody else's imperfect knowledge. [1977]

(In Erickson, 1980, Vol. I, chap. 4, p. 114)

Every time I demonstrate something before a professional audience, I tell them, "Now you didn't see, you didn't hear, you didn't think. These are the steps." It is so much easier to think there is something special about me than to learn to really observe and think. "Erickson is mystical," they say.

(Erickson & Rossi, 1981, p. 249)

You haven't been very attentive because I've been going in and out of a trance while I have been talking to you. I've learned how to go into a trance and I can discuss something with you and watch that rug rise up to this level. (Erickson gestures.)... I can go in and out of a trance without any of you knowing it.

(Zeig, 1980, p. 191)

You see, you didn't listen.

(Zeig, 1980, p. 70)

"And so, walk around with a blank face, your mouth shut, your eyes open and your ears open, and you wait to form your judgement until you have some actual evidence to support your inferences and your judgements."

(Zeig, 1980, p. 234)

One's appreciation of, and understanding of the normal or the usual is requisite for any understanding of the abnormal or the unusual. [1977]

(In Erickson, 1980, Vol. II, chap. 18, p. 179)

Anybody doing therapy ought to get to know the range of human behavior.

(Erickson & Rossi, 1981, p. 86)

You must observe ordinary behavior and be perfectly willing to use it.

(Erickson & Rossi, 1981, p. 17)

I knew that you would because everybody else does it!

(Erickson & Rossi, 1981, p. 231)

And you work with patients and you work with your understanding and your understandings come from your knowledge of how you behave. In your observations of the behavior of others you need to have a vivid observation of your own past behavior.

(Erickson, Rossi & Rossi, 1976, p. 289)

Kay Thompson (1975) has reported to me that Milton summed up the essence of good therapy in another single word which I consider equally valid, and that is the command: "Observe!"

(Beahrs, 1977, p. 60)

And therefore you have to have an open mind; not a critical mind, not a judgemental mind, but a curious, a scientific mind wondering what the real situation is. And so you try to appraise it.

(ASCH, 1980, Taped Lecture, 7/16/65)

The wider your understandings of human nature, the biological processes, the history of individual living, the wider your knowledge of your own reactions, of your own potentials, the better you will practice and the better you will live.

(ASCH, 1980, Taped Lecture, 7/16/65)

I think it is tremendously important that you observe everything that's possible and then if you want to use hypnosis you know how to verbalize your suggestions to influence your patient, to elicit their responses.

(ASCH, 1980, Taped Lecture, 7/16/65)

And if you observe a large number of people carefully, you will learn to recognize that.

(Zeig, 1980, p. 161)

When you look at things, look at them.

(Zeig, 1980, p. 169)

And if you learn to observe, you can learn to recognize those changes almost immediately.

(Zeig, 1980, p. 233)

That's why it's so necessary to observe subjects over and over and over again.

(Zeig, 1980, p. 351)

Now the next thing I want to stress is this. For heaven's sakes look at your patient. *Really see* your patient.

(ASCH, 1980, Taped Lecture, 7/16/65)

You meet, you observe your patient — get acquainted with them. To recognize the little things, the little bit of behavior that they're manifesting.

(ASCH, 1980 Taped Lecture, 7/16/65)

My task was that of observing the patient and working with him. [1966]

(In Erickson, 1980, Vol. II, chap. 34, p. 352)

I looked very carefully for everything.
(Zeig, 1980, p. 285)

I'm training him (Dr. Rossi) in observation.
(Erickson & Rossi, 1981, p.107)

Whenever I made an observation, I wrote it down, sealed it in an envelope and put it in a drawer. Sometime later, when I made another observation, I'd write it down, and then compare it with the first observation I made.
(Zeig, 1980, p. 159)

To begin, my first procedure was to make a visual and auditory survey of the interview situation. I wanted to know what my patient could see and hear and how a shift of his gaze or a change of his position would change the object content of his visual field. I also was interested in the various sounds, probable, possible, and inclusive of street noises, that could intrude upon the situation. [1964]
(In Erickson, 1980, Vol. II, chap. 34, p. 352)

I noticed that licking of her lips, the directing of her glance, her general body movements. [1959]
(In Erickson, 1980, Vol. I, chap. 9, p. 222)

I had always been interested in anthropology, and I think anthropology should be something all psychotherapists should read and know about, because different ethnic groups have different ways of thinking about things.
(Zeig, 1980, p. 119)

If you observe children you learn they do this sort of thing all the time. [1976]

(In Erickson, 1980, Vol. I, chap. 21, p. 441)

With my eight children, I've watched each one of them discover their own physical identity. They all follow the same general pattern.

(Zeig, 1980, p. 236)

Don't look at your peers or your family. That's an unwarranted intrusion into the privacy of others.

(Zeig, 1980, p. 161)

When you look at your peers or your family, your own innate sense of courtesy and privacy will stop you from learning.

(Zeig, 1980, p. 162)

I will read faces and if any of you dislike me, I'll know it.

(Zeig, 1980, p. 162)

When a woman begins her sex life, it's a biological function of her body, and all of her body becomes involved. As soon as she begins having sex regularly, her hairline is likely to change slightly, her eyebrow ridges become a millimeter longer, her chin gets a little bit heavier, her lips a little bit thicker, the angle of the jaw changes, the calcium content of the spine changes, the center of gravity changes, breasts and fat pads of the hips become either larger or denser.

(Zeig, 1980, p. 161)

Years ago I'd write out about 40 pages of suggestions that I would condense down to 20 pages and then down to 10. Then I'd carefully reformulate and make good use of every word and phrase so I'd finally condense it down to about five pages. Everyone who is serious about learning suggestion needs to go through that process to become truly aware of just what they are really saying. [1976-1978]

(In Erickson, 1980, Vol. 1, chap. 23, p. 489)

I want you to notice how connected everything is even though its all impromptu. *It is a language I've learned, a careful study. I know all the articles of speech and I know the meanings of all the words. Because I learned it carefully, I can speak it easily.*

(Erickson & Rossi, 1979, p. 295)

Nobody seemed to understand my questions about breathing. Soon I began to keep my inquiries to myself, since everybody dismissed them as foolish.
This only enhanced my curiosity. [1960's]

(In Erickson, 1980, Vol. 1, chap. 16, p. 363)

Summary

By observing himself and others carefully and objectively throughout his lifetime, Erickson was able to notice things that most of us overlook. He noticed how much people learn and know but forget that they have learned and do not realize that they know. He noticed that people continuously give off and respond to stimuli or communications that occur outside their conscious awareness. He noticed how vast, creative, and orderly are the potential patterns of human thought and behavior and how effectively they are limited and restricted in particular ways by cultural values and by individual experiences. He noticed how unobservant most people are and how many assumptions they impose upon the reality around them. These and other observations formed the foundation for his understanding of people and became the "facts" that guided his hypnotic and psychotherapeutic interventions. Everything he did hypnotically and psychotherapeutically was derived from what he perceived about the particular patient with whom he was working and from what he already knew about people in general from his previous observations.

Thus, everything contained in the remainder of this book, including Erickson's general descriptions of human functioning, his definitions, and his hypnotherapeutic guidelines, rests firmly upon the bedrock of his intelligent critical observation. This point cannot be repeated too often because it is essential to an appreciation of what he had to offer. Only when we stop trying to construct theoretical models or to impose our previously learned constructs upon his words and instead accept what he is saying as a direct description of what *is*, can we effectively comprehend or utilize his wisdom. There is nothing in his words to figure out, though the temptation to do so is overwhelming. There is only a fascinating and humbling description of what people do and of how they can learn to do those things more effectively.

Erickson's general descriptions of human behavior and his guidelines for using what people are and can do will facilitate the process of becoming a more effective hypnotist, therapist, or individual. If we are to follow in Erickson's footsteps we must do more than simply feed upon those of his observations that we can locate and understand; we must obey his injunction to *observe* and examine everything about ourselves and others over and over again in increasingly fine detail. Erickson provided us with a map of the human territory, but eventually we must explore it ourselves in order to develop an accurate picture of it, a feeling for it, and an ability to function effectively within it.

CHAPTER TWO

THE CONSCIOUS MIND

Erickson's observations regarding the basic nature of people eventually led him to a set of general conclusions regarding the conscious and the unconscious minds. This dichotomy apparently served as a shorthand summary for him, a means by which he was able to capture a vast amount of accumulated information within two relatively simple concepts. Even a brief review of his publications suggests that an understanding of the information contained within this dichotomy is necessary for a useful comprehension of his subsequent comments regarding the techniques of psychotherapy and hypnosis. This chapter, therefore, will review the developmental basis and nature of the conscious mind, Chapter 3 will present a description of the unconscious mind, and Chapter 4 will analyze the potential pathological consequences of their functioning and interactions. This observationally based information will then be used as a background for a presentation of his descriptions of the purpose and process of hypnosis and psychotherapy.

Every Person is Unique

One of the most fundamental conclusions drawn by Erickson after his years of observation was that every individual is unique. People differ physiologically and even perceptually. They react differently to the same stimuli and they develop unique personalities as a result.

Erickson's admiration and respect for the qualities specific to each individual prevented him from trying to impose any particular attitudes or behaviors upon his patients and convinced him that no single theory could ever describe all people accurately. He was willing to acknowledge that careful observation of individuals could reveal a pattern or trend of human beings in general and it is this general trend that will be described in the following pages. But he was unwilling to accept the possibility that anyone could ever actually understand, explain, or describe the unique expression of that pattern in any specific person. The best we can hope to do, he maintained, is to develop an appreciation for the general qualities of people and to use that general appreciation as a guidepost in our observations of each individual's particular expression of those general qualities. People behave in accord with their own patterns and they must be responded to with a recognition of their unique individuality. To do otherwise is to impose artificial and arbitrary constraints upon them as individuals, something that Erickson believed patients would justifiably resist.

I think we all should know that every individual is unique... There are no duplicates. In the three and one-half million years that man has lived on earth, I think I am quite safe in saying there are no duplicate fingerprints, no duplicate individuals. Fraternal twins are very,

very different in their fingerprints, their resistance to disease, their psychological structure and personality.

(Zeig, 1980, p. 104)

And so far as I've found in 50 years, every person is a different individual. I always meet every person as an individual, emphasizing his or her own individual qualities.

(Zeig, 1980, p. 220)

Every patient who comes in to you represents a different personality, a different attitude, a different background of experience.

(Haley, 1967, p. 534)

I think any theoretically based psychotherapy is mistaken because each person is different.

(Zeig, 1980, p. 131)

No person can really understand the individual patterns of learning and response of another. [1952]

(In Erickson, 1980, Vol. I, chap. 6, p. 154)

Although each individual is unique in all of his experiential life, single instances often illustrate clearly and vividly aspects and facts of general configurations, trends and patterns. Rather than proof of specific ideas, an illustration or portrayal of possibilities is often the proper goal of experimental work.

(Erickson, 1953, p. 2)

The need to appreciate the subject as a person possessing individuality which must be respected cannot be overemphasized. Such appreciation and respect constitute a foundation for recognizing and differentiating conscious and unconscious behavior. [1952]

(In Erickson, 1980, Vol. I, chap. 6, p. 146)

The Primary Joy of Life is Freedom

Erickson believed that freedom or self-determination, being able to do what you want to do, is one of the primary pleasures of life. Being inept, confused, or unnecessarily constrained creates a lack of freedom and a lack of freedom is something everyone necessarily resists, tries to avoid, or reacts to with discomfort.

> **It might be well to keep in mind the small child's frequent demonstration of the right to self-determination.**
> *(Erickson, 1954a, p. 173)*

> **A small child always asks, "Can I do it when I want to?" The feeling of comfort and freedom is very important.**
> *(Erickson & Rossi, 1979, p. 215)*

> **If you tell anyone they *have* to do something, they invariably come back with they *don't*.**
> *(Erickson & Rossi, 1979, p. 253)*

> **When you are duty bound, you don't like it.**
> *(Zeig, 1980, p. 317)*

> **And I was really doing it! And what greater joy is there than doing what you want to do? [1977]**
> *(In Erickson, 1980, Vol. I, chap. 4, p. 130)*

> **I always find when I can do something, it's pleasurable. [1977]**
> *(In Erickson, 1980, Vol. I, chap. 4, p. 130)*

> **If you are uncertain about yourself, you can't be certain about anything else.**
> *(Erickson, Rossi & Rossi, 1967, p. 106)*

Anything is better than that state of doubt.
(Erickson, Rossi & Rossi, 1976, p. 106)

If the surrounding reality becomes unclear, they want it cleared up by being told something.
(Erickson, Rossi & Rossi, 1976, p. 107)

Since it is awfully uncomfortable to lose reality, you have to replace that reality with another.
(Erickson, Rossi & Rossi, 1976, p. 87)

If you are uncertain about something, you tend to avoid it.
(Erickson, Rossi & Rossi, 1976, p. 106)

You know, ordinarily, what is what about yourself and the other person. When confused you suddenly become concerned about who you are and the other person seems to be fading.
(Erickson, Rossi & Rossi, 1976, p. 106)

In real life, as one grows up through puberty, one naturally goes through periods of great uncertainty; believing and unbelieving.
(Erickson, Rossi & Rossi, 1976, p. 185)

But everybody likes to put together things that belong together. [1977]
(In Erickson, 1980, Vol. I, chap. 21, p. 435)

Experience is the Source of Learning

The initial obstacle confronted by the child in its pursuit of freedom through mastery is its lack of experience. Mastery and understanding, even the simple act of perceiving, all require a history of experiences in that arena. The child lacks experience, its only source of learning and knowing; hence it lacks knowledge and freedom. But it has a tremendous capacity to accumulate experiences, to decipher them, and to utilize them. The human infant is endowed with a brain composed of billions of interactive nerve cells that continually receive information from many diverse sources. These complex quantities of stimuli must be organized and deciphered if mastery is to begin. Thus the child's first order of business probably is to learn how to focus its attention upon, to become aware of, or to respond selectively to *one* kind of input at a time. In other words, it probably must begin with a mastery of its attentional processes.

Actually, as Erickson noted, no one really knows what a child learns first. But it seems evident that every child must, of necessity, first orient itself largely toward the realities of its senses and its body. The child must learn to focus its attention upon sights, sounds, and tastes. It must learn where its hands and arms are and how to move them. It must learn to walk, to talk, and to think.

> **And you need to realize in each first experience, not knowing prevents us from noticing even though we do record.**
>
> *(Erickson & Rossi, 1979, p. 308)*

> **This uncertain bobbing up and down, trial and error, is typical of all learnings. You try to do something new, but there are many partial and abortive efforts.**
>
> *(Erickson & Rossi, 1981, p. 78)*

> **Early learning is a long, hard task, and all kids go through that.**
>
> *(Erickson & Rossi, 1981, p. 187)*

You don't learn all at once. You learn in segmented fashion.

(Erickson & Rossi, 1981, p. 93)

Experience can be very informative.

(Erickson & Rossi, 1981, p. 92)

Experience is the only teacher. [1952]

(In Erickson, 1980, Vol. I, Chapter 6, p. 148)

We really don't know what any one person learns first.

(Erickson & Rossi, 1981, p. 198)

There was a time when you didn't even know you were a people.

(Erickson & Rossi, 1979, p. 231)

One of the important things you learn when you are first born... is that you don't know you've got a body.

(Zeig, 1980, p. 41)

Now, one thing about a child is that he is unacquainted with his body. He doesn't know that his hands are his. He doesn't know that he is moving them. He doesn't recognize his knees or his feet. They are just objects. So he has to feel them over and over again. And learning to recognize your body is really a very difficult thing.

(Zeig, 1980, p. 236)

One time you didn't know those were your hands, so you tried to pick up your right hand with your right hand.

(Erickson & Rossi, 1979, p. 231)

And little Johnny has to locate and identify every part of his body.

(Zeig, 1980, p. 238)

I have personally experienced polio, and I know something about the things that can happen to a person who has had polio. You can forget your body, you can lose your awareness of the various parts of your body. [1960]

(In Erickson 1980, Vol. II, chap. 31, p. 323)

It took a long, long time for me to learn where my feet were, and to recognize the individual parts of my body.

(Zeig, 1980, p. 236)

So the relative distance to various parts of the body differs almost from day to day — at least from week to week.

(Zeig, 1980, p. 238)

He has to know it from the front, from below, from above and from in back. Then he is secure in his knowledge.

(Zeig, 1980, p. 237)

The Importance of Expectation and Reward

Learning is a difficult and complex process at best, one that always involves some pain, failure, and risk, and people can be lazy beings who tend to avoid pain or difficulties whenever possible. Accordingly, people must hope or expect to succeed eventually or they may refuse to try or may give up too soon. Similarly, their successes must be recognized or acknowledged for the same reason. Children are no different from adults in this respect, and many children seem to fail to learn things simply because their parents do not expect them to do so, do not recognize their strides in that direction or do not motivate them effectively.

Most children are expected to be able to learn how to walk and most do a reasonably good job of mastering their muscles. The motivation to do so seems to be quite intrinsic and intense. They usually do such a good job, in fact, that eventually they can pay less and less attention to these overlearned activities and can turn their conscious attention instead to the environment, with which their mobility has brought them increased contact.

All I did was give a look of confident expectation. Now that's the important thing. An infant learning to walk, you know he can learn to walk, but the infant doesn't know. You give the infant the confident support of your expectation.

(Erickson, Rossi & Rossi, 1976, p. 282)

Similarly, respect must be given to the child's ideational comprehension with no effort to derogate or minimize the child's capacity to understand. It is better to expect too great a comprehension than to offend by implying a deficiency. [1958]

(In Erickson, 1980, Vol. IV, chap. 15, p. 176)

Full regard must be given to the human need to succeed and to the desire for recognition by the self and others of that success. [1952]

(In Erickson, 1980, Vol. I, chap. 6, p. 151)

Deeds are the offspring of hope and expectancy.

(Erickson, 1954c, p. 261)

People always have that tendency to put off working on a problem to tomorrow.

(Erickson, Rossi & Rossi, 1976, p. 196)

People can be lazy. If I started teaching by precision, I'd bore them.

(Zeig, 1980, p. 354)

And one usually starts with rather simple things. Because human beings are essentially, fundamentally, rather simple creatures.

(Erickson & Rossi, 1981, p. 12)

Now another thing that you ought to bear in mind is this matter of escape reactions. What do you do when something painful comes along? You want to escape from it.

(ASCH, 1980, Taped Lecture, 7/18/65)

Yes. People like to escape from things. You'd better bear that in mind. And their escape is a very generalized reaction. And so the question is "How much escape do they really want?" And bear in mind that normally, naturally we have a wealth of ways of escaping that are normal and that hypnotically you can use the same mechanisms.

(ASCH, 1980, Taped Lecture, 7/16/65)

Integrating With Reality

Mastery of the basic physiological equipment occurs fairly rapidly even though it is a complex and difficult process. Mastery of and effective functioning within the external physical and social environment, however, is a much more challenging process requiring constant vigilance and continual learning throughout one's life.

People, as a consequence, ordinarily have their conscious awareness rather diffusely focused upon external realities. They must scan one thing after another if they are to monitor the complex variety of events around them. Unless they are aware of the significant events and processes occurring around them, they will be unable to respond in those self-protective or self-enhancing ways that promote freedom and survival. Hence their awareness flits from this to that in a continual scanning of internal and external circumstances.

However, awareness of events by itself is insufficient. The *meaning* of those events must be determined on the basis of the ever-increasing accumulation of experientially based learnings acquired by the child. Events must be understood, not just noticed, if the child is to determine to what to respond and how to respond to it. Furthermore, the simpler and more painless this understanding is, the more likely the child is to acquire it. Parsimony is not just a scientific preference.

> You tend to orient to reality and to give your attention in a diffuse way. [1959]
>
> *(In Erickson, 1980, Vol. III, chap. 4, p. 28)*

> Now the conscious mind is your state of immediate awareness. Consciously, you are aware of the wheelchair, the rug on the floor, the other people present, the lights, the bookcases, the night-blooming cacti flowers, the pictures on the wall, Count Dracula on the wall right behind you. ("Count Dracula" is a dried skate that hangs on one wall.) In other words, you are dividing your attention between what I say and everything around you.
>
> *(Zeig, 1980, p. 33)*

> In the ordinary state of conscious awareness, however, we are constantlly orienting ourselves to the concrete reality around us. We do this as a matter of biological preservation... You remain well aware of these facts, and from moment to moment you reinforce this orientation to reality. [1960]
>
> *(In Erickson, 1980, Vol. II, chap. 31, p. 321)*

People in the nontrance state do not lose complete general awareness of the immediate reality surroundings nor of the general context of thinking and speaking; and should they do so in partial fashion, they "come to" with a start, explaining (usually without a request to do so), "For a moment or two there I absentmindedly forgot everything except what I was thinking," reorienting themselves as they speak to their general environment. But it is to the actual reality that they orient themselves. [1967]

(In Erickson, 1980, Vol. I, chap. 2, p. 40)

In the ordinary waking state, however, it appears that the responsive functioning occurs in relationship to the stimulus as emerging from, and constituting only a part of, a much greater and seemingly more significant reality background. [1958]

(In Erickson, 1980, Vol. II, chap. 19, p. 194)

Waking responsiveness tends to be goal-directed towards an integration with objective reality in some form. [1958]

(In Erickson, 1980, Vol. II, chap. 19, p. 192)

Learning the Constraints of Reality

Obviously, absolute freedom is an impossibility because reality imposes restrictions, limitations, and consequences that cannot or should not be ignored. The process of growth and development, therefore, is the process of learning what those limitations, restrictions, and possibilities are.

Thus, the newborn infant is confronted with a monumental task. In order to navigate freely within its environment, and yet to be so well integrated into the environment that it will survive, it must learn how to attend to, to decipher and to utilize the tremendously complex influx of sensations from its senses in a way that enhances its purposes and goal attainments. It must accumulate organized memories of previous experiences and develop an understanding of the rules of reality from them. It must learn how to control its muscles and it must learn what its own abilities and weaknesses are. In short, it must develop an organized view of its internal and external environments and it must learn how to respond appropriately and freely within the constraints and rules of those environments.

In the process of living, the price of survival is eternal vigilance and the willingness to learn. The sooner one becomes aware of realities and the sooner one adjusts to them, the quicker is the process of adjustment and the happier the experience of living. When one knows the boundaries, restrictions and limitations that govern, then he is free to utilize satisfactorily whatever is available. [1962]

(In Erickson, 1980, Vol. IV, chap. 57, p. 514)

Reality, security, and the definition of boundaries and limitations constitute important considerations in the growth of understanding in childhood. To an eight year old child, the question of what constitutes power and strength and reality and security can be a serious matter. When one is small, weak, and intelligent, living in an undefined world of intellectual and emotional fluctuations, one seeks to learn what is really strong, secure, and safe. [1962]

(In Erickson, 1980, Vol. IV, chap. 57, p. 507)

Reality, security, definition of boundaries and limitations all constitute important considerations in the childhood growth of understandings. There is a desperate need to reach out and to define one's self and others. [1975]

(In Erickson, 1980, Vol. I, chap. 20, p. 419)

There governs children, as growing, developing organisms, an ever-present motivation to seek for more and better understandings of all that is about them. [1958]

(In Erickson, 1980, Vol. IV, chap. 15, p. 174)

Children have a driving need to learn and to discover, and every stimulus constitutes, for them, a possible opportunity to respond in some new way. [1958]

(In Erickson, 1980, Vol. IV, chap. 15, p. 174)

Building a Frame of Reference

As the child interacts with its environment and gains experience, it gradually builds an overall view of its reality context. At first, this context is objectively based (though naive) and fairly fluid. The child lacks experience but is open to new information that will improve its understanding.

Reality, however, is enormously complex and difficult to observe or to analyze effectively. Because people tend to avoid difficult or painful circumstances or to transform them into simpler and more pleasing ones, most children will accept shorter, easier, more straightforward descriptions of reality if they are offered. Adults provide these shorthand versions of reality in the form of arbitrary classification systems, attitudes, beliefs, theories, culturally based rules of conduct, and even a predefined categorization and naming system called language.

Because each child is physiologically unique and has unique experiences, the shorthand rules or images of reality eventually adopted by each individual will be relatively unique as well. Once the child has picked up the general rules and principles that the members of its culture have agreed to use, it will begin applying these general rules in its own unique manner and will develop a unique model of reality.

Over time the child constructs an increasingly well-organized shorthand view or model of reality through which the world is viewed and analyzed. This model of reality enables the child to understand the meaning of events quickly and easily and also allows it to determine quickly what appears to be an appropriate response. The objective direct view of reality is gradually replaced by the simpler, more straightforward (though less accurate) conscious model. The complex, demanding, and time-consuming qualities of objective observation and analysis make this development of a shorthand model appealing and adaptive. Even adults opt for simple theories and universally applicable techniques although careful observation of complex circumstances might eventually provide a more accurate awareness and a more effective response.

The accumulated shorthand model or context of understandings that acts as a filter between the person's conscious awareness and objective reality and that subsequently dictates the meaning of events and provides the organizations for responses *is what Erickson referred to as the conscious mind.* Almost everything an individual thinks, perceives and does at a conscious level of awareness is a reflection of or is influenced by this conscious frame of reference.

> **Children are small, young people. As such, they define the world and its events in a different way than does the adult, and their experiential learnings are limited and quite different from those of the adult. [1958]**
> *(In Erickson, 1980, Vol. IV, chap. 15, p. 174)*

Children have their own ideas and need to have them respected, but they are readily open to any modification of those ideas intelligently presented to them. [1958]
(In Erickson, 1980, Vol. IV, chap. 15, p. 176)

And philosophers of old have said, "As a man thinketh, he is."
(Erickson & Rossi, 1979, p. 262)

And all philosophers say, reality is all in the head.
(Zeig, 1980, p. 90)

A central consideration in the proposed experimental project was suggested by the well known Biblical saying, "As a man thinketh in his heart, so is he." [1964]
(In Erickson, 1980, Vol. I, chap. 1, p. 4)

Waking subjects are restricted to their general conscious concepts of how to function intellectually. [1962]
(In Erickson, 1980, Vol. III, chap. 13, p. 117)

Because consciously you behave in accord with the conscious universe, the conscious patterns of behavior.
(ASCH, 1980, Taped Lecture, 2/2/66)

The subjects accept those ideas in terms of their own frames of reference and a lifetime of experiential learning. These experiential learnings may be unusual and quite unexpected. [1960]
(In Erickson, 1980, Vol. II, chap. 31, p. 313)

Language Development

At first a child's conscious understandings or framework can be expressed only behaviorally through the organization of its responses to its environment. Eventually, however, these experientially acquired understandings of the conscious mind begin to be influenced by and expressed within a language system. Learning to understand language and to speak is a slow, trial-and-error process just as most learning seems to be. It is also an individual-specific process in the sense that every person develops unique experientially based definitions or meanings for each word. Thus, for example, the word "mother" conjures up a slightly different set of associations and responses for each person — usually associations derived from the unique patterns of interaction with the person's own mother. Every word has a unique implication or meaning for each individual that stems from and defines their unique frame of reference.

A newly born baby is extremely ignorant. It has a sucking reflex and it can cry. But it is a meaningless cry. It is, I expect, the discomfort with the new environment.

(Zeig, 1980, p. 234)

After a while, mother begins to notice that the meaningless cries acquire a meaning.

(Zeig, 1980, p. 235)

Each cry is altered as the child begins to comprehend various things.

(Zeig, 1980, p. 235)

There's another thing to be taken into consideration: how all of us learn to talk. There's a long, long experience of making errors... There's a wealth of learning you get from making mistakes.

(Zeig, 1980, p. 336)

The problem in learning to speak well is in your willingness to learn slowly.

(Erickson & Rossi, 1981, p. 82)

We always translate the other person's language into our own language.

(Zeig, 1980, p. 64)

Because when you talk to people, they hear you in their language.

(Zeig, 1980, p. 70)

I had to wait until I understood *her* words.

(Zeig, 1980, p. 158)

You o ght to be acquainted with the linguistic patterns of your patients. And we all have our own personal understandings.

(Zeig, 1980, p. 78)

All of you will apply what I say in accordance with your own specific understandings.

(Zeig, 1980, p. 64)

Now, every word in any language has usually a lot of different meanings.

(Zeig, 1980, p. 78)

Rigidity and Non-objectivity of Conscious Frames of Reference

At first the ordinary person's mind or brain is relatively unstructured, objective, flexible, and open to new learnings. Over time, however, it naturally becomes increasingly rigid, biased, idiosyncratic, and unable to accept perceptions, learnings, or responses that cannot be accommodated by its previously adopted structure. Increases in "understanding" or the acceptance and utilization of specific culturally imposed conscious frames of reference necessarily leads to less flexibility and more tightly organized perceptions and responses. Eventually the entire conscious awareness of the individual may become restrictively governed or dictated by the very structure that originally developed to allow an increased freedom of response. Obviously, the degree of rigidity and bias of conscious frames of reference will vary from person to person and from culture to culture but the general trend is in the direction of increased organization and rigidity of structure.

> Now, Dr. Rossi here is somebody who is trained in psychology. He has been oriented to place individual meanings or interpretation on everything according to his past teachers. *He does not know very much about* looking at or *experiencing reality*. He must experience reality in terms of what he has been taught and read.
>
> *(Erickson & Rossi, 1981, p. 193)*

> The author has encountered such rigidity of frames of reference. [1967]
>
> *(Erickson, 1980, Vol. I, chap. 2, p. 38)*

> These are all conscious biases. You can broaden your activity, however, if you recognize the bias. Experimentalists in hypnosis ought to know about the unlimited number of biases that everybody builds up.
>
> *(Erickson, Rossi & Rossi, 1976, p. 179)*

> Biases are a part of our conscious living.
>
> *(Erickson, Rossi & Rossi, 1976, p. 180)*

> **They are not just biases, they are part of the way we
> experience the world.**
> *(Erickson, Rossi & Rossi, 1976, p. 180)*

> **When you use the word "bias" it is so easily
> misunderstood. It is actually a *common set.***
> *(Erickson, Rossi & Rossi, 1976, p. 180)*

> **I want to make her aware that she has many many
> rigid sets. Everybody has.**
> *(Erickson, Rossi & Rossi, 1976, p. 213)*

> **People say, "But I always eat cereal for breakfast! But
> we always have chicken on Sunday." These are all con-
> scious biases.**
> *(Erickson, Rossi & Rossi, 1976, pp. 178–179)*

> **A young man says, "It's a nice day today." His frame
> of reference is a picnic with his sweetheart. A farmer
> says, "It's a nice day today." His frame of reference is
> that it is a good day to mow hay... Totally different
> meanings, yet you could understand them when you
> knew their frame of reference.**
> *(Erickson & Rossi, 1981, p. 255)*

Complexity of Conscious Frames of Mind

As the child grows older it moves into new settings and
situations which often place the child in totally new contexts
of demands and expectations. In essence, the child is confronted by new realities. Such circumstances often dictate the
development of somewhat new and different conscious frames
of reference. Consequently, over time the conscious mind may
develop a number of separate frameworks or perspectives,
each of which may be utilized in special circumstances in

response to special contextual demands. Usually these various frameworks are coherently organized or interrelated and aspects of one may blend into or even become the foundation for another. In some sense they each usually represent variations on a basic underlying theme rather than a totally separate or unique perspective. Subjectively the individual experiences a smooth and almost automatic transition from one perspective to another as the external circumstances change and conscious awareness shifts from one perspective or filter to another. However, when one of these conscious frameworks of perception, thought, or response contains something completely unacceptable to the others it may become completely severed or isolated from the rest of the conscious mind, a phenomenon seen at various times in true multiple personalities.

As the complex structure of the whole conscious mind becomes more tightly or completely organized, it becomes an increasingly distinct and exclusive set of patterns of perception, thought, and response. The brain remains capable of numerous other patterns and may engage in them at times, but if events or thoughts do not "fit" into the acceptable patterns of the structure of the adopted conscious mind, then they usually are excluded from consideration and do not become available to the person who is aware only of those things allowed through the filter of the conscious mind. The conscious mind, therefore, eventually becomes a dissociated, unique, and complex entity that provides rather specific, exclusive views and ways of thinking about the world.

The human personality is characterized by infinite varieties and complexities of development and organization, and it is not a simple limited unitary organization. It is, rather, to be regarded as having as complicated a

structure, organization, and development as has the individual's experiential background. [circa 1940's]
(In Erickson, 1980, Vol. III, chap. 24, p.262)

There can be separate states of awareness that develop spontaneously in ordinary life. [circa 1940's]
(In Erickson, 1980, Vol. III, chap. 8, p. 61)

From this realization of the complexity of the structure of the personality there has developed the understanding of the possibility — and the actual probability — of separate and specific integrations within the total organization as a common characteristic...In this regard Oberndorf has spoken of "that galaxy of personalities which constitute the individual." [circa 1940's]
(In Erickson, 1980, Vol. III, Chap. 24, p. 263)

Nor is there as yet sufficient evidence at hand to establish how many degrees of such multiple formations may exist. [1939]
(In Erickson, 1980, Vol. III, chap. 23, p. 256)

In fact one must ask whether one is justified in dismissing the possibility that all acts of repression involve the creation of a larval form of a secondary personality. [1939]
(In Erickson, 1980, Vol. III, chap. 23, pp. 256 — 257)

So little has been said about the varying role of the patient who may present to the analyst not one personality but many. [1939]
(In Erickson, 1980, Vol. III, chap. 23, p. 256)

Summary

All unique individuals attempt to maintain their freedom to respond by extending their awareness and understanding of the nature of the rules of their reality. Their slowly accumulated, experientially, and culturally based conscious frame of reference eventually provides the understanding of what can or should be done and these understandings guide their responses. As long as their awareness is directed toward the world through that frame of reference, perspective, set or state of mind, all thoughts, perceptions, and responses are influenced, limited, or directed by it.

CHAPTER THREE

THE UNCONSCIOUS MIND

It is unfortunate, perhaps, that so much of what Erickson observed and knew about human functioning was reduced to a shorthand reference to the unconscious and the conscious. In spite of his frequent declarations that this bifurcation of people into conscious and unconscious levels of functioning was a "conceptual convenience," it is potentially a very confusing and misleading oversimplification. Not only does the term "unconscious" carry a host of undesirable and inaccurate connotations from numerous theoretical systems, the conscious-unconscious duality itself fails to convey adequately Erickson's complex understanding of human personality.

The term "unconscious," for example, conjures up Freudian and Jungian implications for most of us almost automatically, none of which have any relevance to Erickson's observations at all. Even when these traditional theoretical connotations are overcome, there remains the problem of eliminating the implied mystical notions of an all-knowing, infallible unconscious and other everyday interpretations related to the process of being "knocked unconscious" by a blow to the head or by drugs. As a careful review of the material presented in this chapter should suggest, none of these uses of the term are relevant to what Erickson meant by the "unconscious."

Erickson was not unaware of these potential sources of conceptual confusion. Early in his career he sometimes substituted the term subconscious and often put the term unconscious in quotes in an apparent attempt to suggest an idiosyncratic definition. On later occasions he referred instead to "a different level of awareness," to "one's own actual potentialities," and to "useful unrealized self-knowledge." Generally, however, he simply used the term "unconscious" without specific qualification, although it must be reemphasized that what he meant by the term "unconscious" was something vastly different from what most authors have meant by it. A genuine appreciation for what he had to offer requires the adoption of his understandings and the avoidance of imposed assumptions.

The unwarranted and misleading implications of the term "unconscious" are not the only roadblocks to a comprehension of the fundamental concepts underlying Erickson's approach. As indicated earlier, the conscious-unconscious dichotomy itself also is a potential source of confusion. Aside from the unavoidable fact that it almost necessarily leads some people into a questionable application of the right-left hemisphere paradigm that is now being used to account for almost all dichotomous human behavior, it also fails to capture the complexity of human functioning that Dr. Erickson actually observed. Multiple levels of awareness, information processing and responding from within a multitude of conceptual conscious and unconscious frameworks or perspectives were apparent to him. Care must be taken, therefore, to avoid confusing this "conceptual convenience" with a completely accurate description of reality. Although accurate as far as it goes, Erickson saw many more dimensions to people than this dichotomy implies.

Having prefaced this presentation with what may seem to be an inordinate number of qualifications or cautions, an attempt now will be made to summarize or to review the term "unconscious" from Erickson's perspective.

The Reality of the Unconscious

It is important at the outset to recognize that when Erickson referred to the unconscious mind he was referring to a very real, observable, demonstrable, phenomenon. He was not merely using the term as a metaphor or as a construct. He meant that people actually *have* an unconscious mind or unconsicous levels of awareness in the same sense that they have an arm or a leg. The unconscious, in Erickson's view, is a necessary, observable, and very real component of every human personality.

> Now what I'd like to have you understand is this: that you have a conscious mind, and you know that and I know that, and you have an unconscious mind or subconscious mind, and you know that I mean by that, do you not?
>
> *(Erickson & Rossi, 1981, p. 157)*

> [Hypnosis] is characterized by various physiological concomitants, and by a functioning of the personality at a level of awareness other than the ordinary or usual state of awareness. For convenience in conceptualization, this special state, or level of awareness, has been termed "unconscious" or "subconscious". [1948]
>
> *(In Erickson, 1980, Vol. IV, chap. 4, p. 37)*

> The activity involved in this (i.e. in automatic writing and crystal-gazing) is perhaps one of the best "proofs" of the existence of the "subconscious" mind. [1943]
>
> *(In Erickson, 1980, Vol. III, chap. 1, p. 10)*
>
> Furthermore, the unconscious as such, not as transformed into the conscious, constitutes an essential part of psychological functioning.
>
> *(Erickson, 1953, p.2)*

The Separate Abilities of the Unconscious

Not only is the unconscious real, it also is distinct and separate from the conscious mind. It coexists with the conscious mind as totally separate, mutually exclusive processes of awareness, learning, and response. Its activities continue in parallel with the activities of the conscious mind, although there are influence processes from one system to the other.

The unconscious can listen to or perceive things that the conscious mind ignores. It can think about one thing while the person is consciously thinking about something else. The unconscious has its own separate interests, memories, and understandings. The unconscious can control physical activities without the conscious mind being aware of it and, as a result, it can communicate with others and express ideas that are outside the range of conscious perception or awareness.

Usually, but not always, the processes and activities of the unconscious mind support or extend the activities and desires of the conscious mind. Under the right circumstances, however, the unconscious mind may act in a more or less autonomous manner, expressing its own desires or understandings only and initiating activities that are unrelated to the processes of the conscious frame of reference.

As indicated previously, one of the principal outcomes of

Erickson's careful observations of himself and others was his cumulative appreciation for the fact that people know much more than they are consciously aware that they know, do much more than they are consciously aware that they do, perceive much more than they are consciously aware of perceiving and have a whole variety of intellectual, behavioral, and physiological capacities about which they also are oblivious. His lifetime of observations consistently led him to the conclusions that humans have and continually use a vast reservoir of experientially acquired learnings of which they are largely unaware, have unused or overlooked capacities, potentials and experientially acquired knowledge, and engage in interactions or communication exchanges with no awareness that they are or have done so. Because all of these events and potentials exist outside the range of ordinary conscious awareness, he naturally referred to them as "unconscious" and to the separate system within which they occurred or existed as the "unconscious mind." By definition therefore, the unconscious is all of those elements of our functioning to which we do not pay attention for one reason or another or about which we are consciously unaware.

Thus, the separateness of the unconscious from the conscious and the actuality or reality of the unconscious are almost definitional necessities as well as objectively observable or demonstrable qualities. Like light and dark, the unconscious and the conscious are defined in terms of each other, although in Erickson's perspective this light-dark dichotomy should probably be applied in the reverse of its typical application with the light representing the unconscious instead of the dark. But no matter how this comparison is made, it is clear that the existence in conscious awareness of only selected features of the overall input and activity of the brain as interpreted from within a particular frame of reference or perspective leaves a lot left over to be accounted for. This accounting is the unconscious, a phenomenon which logic dictates and that careful observation demonstrates.

> **Your unconscious knows all about it — probably more than your conscious mind does — and your unconscious mind can keep from you, from your conscious mind, anything it doesn't want you to know consciously.**
> *(Erickson & Lustig, 1975, Vol. 1, p. 9)*

> **Because you are dealing with a person who has both a conscious mind and an unconscious mind.**
> *(Erickson & Rossi, 1981, p. 6)*

> **R: [Rossi] So the conscious and unconscious really are separate systems.**
> **E: [Erickson] Yes, they are separate systems.**
> *(Erickson, Rossi & Rossi, 1976, p. 258)*

> **Yes, I seem to bifurcate the individual into the conscious and unconscious. When I say something, I may say it to the conscious or I may say it to the unconscious.**
> *(Erickson & Rossi, 1981, p. 103)*

> **The first idea I want to impress upon you is one way of thinking about your patients clinically. It is desirable to use this framework because of the ease of concept formation for the patient. I like to regard my patients as having a conscious mind and an unconscious mind. I expect the two of them to be together in the same person, and I expect both of them to be in the office with me. *When I am talking to a person at the conscious level, I expect him to be listening to me at an unconscious level, as well as consciously.***
> *(Erickson & Rossi, 1981, p. 3)*

Also, it became apparent that there were multiple levels of perception and response, not all of which were necessarily at the usual or conscious level of awareness, but were at levels of understanding not recognized by the self, often popularly described as "instinctive" or "intuitive."

(Bandler & Grinder, 1975, Preface, p. viii)

Now you don't really need to listen to me because your unconscious mind will hear me. You can let your conscious mind wander in any direction it wants to.

(Erickson & Rossi, 1981, p. 189)

I know his unconscious is listening. It has to. He's only a few feet away from me, my voice is loud enough. It will!

(Erickson & Rossi, 1981, p. 200)

Your unconscious mind can listen to me without your knowledge and also deal with something else at the same time.

(Erickson, Rossi & Rossi, 1976, p. 38)

The patient's unconscious mind is listening and understanding much better than is possible for his conscious mind. [1966]

(In Erickson, 1980, Vol. IV, chap. 28, p. 277)

I don't know if you have any conscious idea, but always the unconscious mind has its own thoughts. Its own desires.

(Erickson, Rossi & Rossi, 1976, p. 285)

I'm making it apparent here that there are two sets of interests, and the unconscious is going to have its interests.

(Erickson, Rossi & Rossi, 1976, p. 207)

You demonstrate that the conscious can think one way and the unconscious another. You're going to have a chance to see and prove within yourself that they think differently.

(Erickson, Rossi & Rossi, 1976, p. 171)

Your unconscious learned a lot yesterday. It also learned that we could learn a lot without intruding upon the personality.

(Erickson, Rossi & Rossi, 1976, p. 207)

You let them know that they do know a lot more than they realize. They have that knowledge in their unconscious.

(Erickson, 1980, Vol. IV, p. 98)

It is not necessary for you to remember consciously, because your unconscious mind will remember what I say and what it means, and that is what is necessary. [1953]

(In Erickson, 1980, Vol. IV, Chapter 42, p. 376)

Also, it is explained that thinking can be done separately and independently by both the conscious and unconscious mind, but that such thinking need not necessarily be in agreement. [1961]

(In Erickson, 1980, Vol. I, chap. 5, p. 138)

I tell them that no matter how silent they are, their unconscious mind is beginning to think, beginning to understand, that they themselves do not need to know consciously what is going on in their unconscious mind.

(Erickson & Rossi, 1981, p. 18)

Your unconscious can know the answer, but you don't have to know the answer.

(Erickson & Rossi, 1979, p. 203)

It's important for you to realize that your unconscious mind can start a train of thought, and develop it without your conscious knowledge — and reach conclusions, and let your conscious mind become aware of those conclusions.

(Erickson & Lustig, 1975, Vol. 2, p.4)

I wanted your unconscious mind to have the liberty of doing something while your conscious mind was filled with other things.

(Erickson, Rossi & Rossi, 1976, p. 206)

Your unconscious can try anything it wishes. But your conscious mind isn't going to do anything of importance.

(Erickson, Rossi & Rossi, 1976, p. 9)

And it really doesn't matter what your conscious mind does because your unconscious automatically will do just what it needs to.

(Erickson, Rossi & Rossi, 1976, p. 67)

Consciously chosen words, thoughts, and acts can mean more than one thing at a time: their conscious or manifest content on the one hand, and a latent, unconscious content on the other. [1939]

(In Erickson, 1980, Vol. III, chap. 16, p. 156)

They have had a lifetime of experience in which talking is done at a conscious level, and have no realization that talking is possible at a purely unconscious level of awareness. [1952]

(In Erickson, 1980, Vol. I, chap. 6, p. 145)

His unconscious mind can communicate directly and adequately and is free to make whatever communication it wishes, whether by sign language, verbally or in both manners. [1964]

(In Erickson, 1980, Vol. I, chap. 13, p. 309)

It is impressive to see how ready the unconscious seemed to be to communicate with the examiner by means of this accessory sign language of drawing, while at the same time the consciously organized part of the personality was busy recounting other matters. [1938]

(In Erickson, 1980, Vol. III, chap. 17, p. 174)

She was able to execute consciously an act which in itself was fully expressive and complete, but which simultaneously possessed an additional unrecognized significance at another level of mentation. [1937]

(In Erickson, 1980, Vol. III, chap. 16, p. 150)

With another hypnotic subject, it was possible to carry on a written conversation having a conscious import but which was developed entirely in accord with an import known only to the unconscious mind of the subject and to the investigator without the subject becoming aware consciously of the actual nature of the conversation. [1939]

(In Erickson, 1980, Vol. IV, chap. 1, p. 12)

It would seem, therefore, that humorlessly and quite without conscious comic intent the unconscious can use irony, punning, and the technique of the puzzle. In short, the techniques of conscious humor are an earnest and serious matter in unconscious psychic processes. This is particularly disconcerting when weighty and significant problems are treated by means of unconsciously chosen representatives and devices which to our conscious judgements seem ridiculous and trivial. [1937]

(In Erickson, 1980, Vol. III, chap. 16, p. 157)

As in dreams, puns, elisions, plays on words and similar tricks that we ordinarily think of as frivolous, all play a surprising and somewhat disconcerting role in the communication of important and serious feelings... It is ever a source of fresh amazement when the unconscious processes express weighty and troublesome problems in a shorthand which has in it an element of levity. [1940]

(In Erickson, 1980, Vol. III, chap. 18, p. 186)

[This] served to convince me further that people communicate with each other at "breathing" levels of awareness unknown to them. [circa 1960's]

(In Erickson, 1980, Vol. I chap. 16, p. 364)

Communication can be verbal, but it is also quite obvious that there is a great deal of nonverbal communication. Communication can be an angry look, a lovely look — all kinds of looks and all kinds of gestures. [1960]

(In Erickson, 1980, Vol. II, chap. 31, p. 328)

When do you kiss a pretty girl?... When she is ready, not when you are ready. You wait for that undefinable behavior that she manifests. You don't ask a girl for a kiss, but in her presence you just gaze thoughtfully at the mistletoe. You are just being thoughtful. She gets the idea, and she starts thinking about the kiss.

(Erickson & Rossi, 1981, p. 230)

One student can brush back her hair with a deliberateness that says "I hope that son-of-a-bitch reaches the end of the lecture soon." Then there's that unconscious brushing back of the hair that indicates they are attending to you.

(Erickson & Rossi, 1981, p. 70)

Certain patients, while explaining their problems, will unwittingly nod or shake their heads contradictorily to their actual verbalizations. [1961]

(In Erickson, 1980, Vol. I, chap. 5, p. 138)

There stands a baby, dirty face, tousled of hair, runny nose, wet, smelly, dirty, and its face lights up and it toddles to you so happily because it *knows* its a nice baby and *that you will be glad to like it and that you will want to pick it up.* You know what you will do! So does the baby! *You can't help yourself.* ...Beautiful little child, hair combed, clean, neat, in a state of perfection, but its face says, "Who just who on earth would *ever* want to pick me up?" Certainly you don't, you agree with the child, and you want to find the parents and slap them around for mistreating that child, because you don't want to be greeted again, ever again, by that child in that manner.

(Erickson & Rossi, 1979, p. 437)

You are saying that their unconscious mind can now work, and work secretly, without the awareness of the conscious mind.

(Erickson & Rossi, 1981, p. 18)

The unconscious works without your knowledge and that is the way it prefers.

(Erickson & Rossi, 1976, p. 163)

The Unconscious is a Storehouse

Because Erickson's primary goal in hypnosis and therapy was to help others learn how to use their unconscious capacities to resolve their problems and to respond more freely in new ways, it is not surprising that he emphasized the fact that the unconscious represents a reservoir of unrecognized experientially acquired learnings or knowledge. This feature of the unconscious was of primary interest to him therapeutically and he almost invariably described the unconscious in this way.

Erickson was genuinely impressed by how much people know but do not know that they know. Some of this knowledge consists of psychological, emotional, physical, or intellectual information that originally was consciously and intentionally acquired but later dropped out of conscious awareness. The complex learning underlying walking is an example. The learning that was required to begin to walk is unavailable to most adults, even though they continue to utilize and to rely upon it. Other learning can occur without conscious awareness or purpose. People can learn without consciously knowing that they have learned and can use that learning later without recognizing that they are doing so. This significant type of learning can occur because the unconscious is a separate, parallel system of awareness and information processing.

Finally, unconscious learning can be unused. Even though a large proportion of human behavior is unconscious or automatic and most of what we do intentionally or consciously is dependent upon the use of unconsciously held learnings, a tremendous amount of what we have learned and know is never applied or utilized effectively by us because of our conscious repressions and rigidities.

The unconscious mind or level of awareness, therefore, is a vast storehouse of unrecognized, unused or misused memories and learnings, a storehouse that can provide the basic information and learning necessary for psychotherapeutic or hypnotic responses to occur. The unconscious probably already knows what the person's problem is, the source of the problem, and how to alleviate the problem. As such, it obviously is a potentially beneficial ally in many respects.

> Now, the unconscious mind is a vast storehouse of memories, your learnings. It has to be a storehouse because you cannot keep consciously in mind all the things you know. Your unconscious mind acts as a storehouse. Considering all the learning you have acquired in a lifetime, you use the vast majority of them automatically in order to function.
>
> *(Zeig, 1980, p. 173)*

> In hypnosis we utilize the unconscious mind. What do I mean by the unconscious mind? I mean the back of the mind, the reservoir of learning. The unconscious mind constitutes a storehouse. [1959]
>
> *(In Erickson, 1980, Vol. III, chap. 4, p. 27)*

> The body learns a wealth of unconscious psychological, emotional, neurological, and physiological associations and conditionings. These unconscious learnings, repeatedly reinforced by additional life experiences, constitute the source of the potentials that can be employed through hypnosis. [1967]
>
> *(In Erickson, 1980, Vol. IV, chap. 24, p. 238)*

> Common experience has demonstrated repeatedly that unconscious attitudes toward the body can constitute potent factors in many relationships. Learning processes, physical and physiological functioning, and recovery

from illness are, among others, examples of areas in which unrecognized body attitudes may be of vital significance to the individual. [1960]

(In Erickson, 1980, Vol. II, chap. 21, p. 203)

Yet as a result of experiential events of his past life, there has been built up within his body — although all unrecognized — certain psychological, physiological, and neurological learnings, associations, and conditionings that render it possible for pain to be controlled and even abolished. [1967]

(In Erickson, 1980, Vol. IV, chap. 24, p. 237)

Your unconscious does know much more about you than you do. It's got a whole background of years of learning, feeling, thinking, and doing. And all our days we are learning things — learning how.

(Erickson & Lustig, 1975, Vol. 2, p. 3)

Human beings, once they have learned anything, transfer this learning to the forces that govern their bodies. [1959]

(In Erickson, 1980, Vol. III, chap. 4, p. 27)

The next thing I wish to call to your attention is the matter of the experiential learning that we all absorb during a lifetime of experiences. Little children practice walking and getting up and sitting down, lying down, rolling over, using every muscle and action of their extremities and torso. They get acquainted with the various parts of their bodies and learn the full extent of their capabilities. They learn these things so thoroughly that years later, when they are full-grown adults and have forgotten the process through which they learned their actions they will respond promptly when a mosquito lands on any part of their body. [1959]

(In Erickson, 1980, Vol. III, chap. 4, p. 27)

You do a lot of things automatically.
(Zeig, 1980, p. 222)

You see movements without complete conscious awareness in kids all the time.
(Erickson & Rossi, 1981, p. 77)

There is a lot of your behavior you don't know about.
(Zeig, 1980, p. 42)

When you listen to a radio program of music, for instance, if you want to single out the instruments, you don't look at a bright light or thumb through a book. You close your eyes, you unconsciously turn your dominant ear toward the music, and you carefully shut out visible stimuli. If you are holding a cold glass in your hand, you put it down so that the coldness does not divert your attention away from the music. You are not necessarily aware of performing these actions because your unconscious mind has directed their performance. It knows how you can best hear the music.
(Erickson & Rossi, 1981, p. 24)

In the course of living, from infancy on, you acquired knowledge, but you could not keep all that knowledge in the foreground of your mind. In the development of the human being learning in the unconscious became available in any time of need. When you need to feel comfort, you can feel comfort.
(Erickson, Rossi & Rossi, 1976, p. 155)

And that is something you need to teach your patients, when the appropriate time comes to respond with a certain kind of behavior you can do so. You do not have to know consciously that you already know that behavior.
(ASCH, 1980, Taped Lecture, 7/16/65)

Because the important understanding that you need is this, that any knowledge acquired by your unconscious mind is knowledge that you can use at any appropriate time. But you need not necessarily be aware that you have that knowledge until the moment comes to use it. And then you just quite naturally respond with the appropriate behavior.

(ASCH, 1980, Taped Lecture, 7/16/65)

Your body is a lot wiser than you are.

(Zeig, 1980, p. 63)

A child's body tells him how many swallows for a good drink before he has a chance to absorb much of that water.... So you don't need to be more aware of your learning than a child is of the number of swallows of water.

(Erickson & Rossi, 1981, p. 99)

We are usually unaware of all the automatic responses we make on the basis of the locus of sound and the inflections of voice. [1976–1978]

(In Erickson, 1980, Vol. I, chap. 23, p. 481)

You all can walk, yet you really don't know the movements or the processes.

(Zeig, 1980, p. 37)

Joint sensation and kinesthetic memories are as valid as any other kinds of memories. You can substitute them and modify them. I think there is need for a great deal of research on the characteristics of these different types of learnings and memories, the conditions for change, and the way in which they undergo spontaneous alterations during life. [1960]

(In Erickson, 1980, Vol. II, chap. 31, p. 324)

I had long forgotten that, but my unconscious had remembered it.

(Erickson, Rossi & Rossi, 1976, p. 288)

You see, you are never given a course in accent learning, yet you pick up those accents. You don't know you are picking them up, but you are learning them and you learn how to recognize them.

(Zeig, 1980, p. 314)

The Unconscious is Unknown Potentials

Every normal individual enters this world with a neurological and biophysical system capable of perceiving, thinking, and responding in an incredible variety of ways. As discussed in the previous chapter, during growth and development only a fraction of these potential patterns of perception, understanding, and response become actualized within the conscious mind. The remainder remain hidden from view, unused and generally unavailable. A host of mental frames of reference, beliefs, attitudes, understandings, perceptions, somatic and physical response capabilities and emotions are effectively cut off from ordinary conscious awareness and are relegated to the province of the unconscious.

All of the various phenomena or responses that can be manifested during a hypnotic trance are based upon abilities normally excluded from conscious awareness. A good hypnotic subject is merely a person who has learned how to accept and to use these unconscious capacities. Hypnosis does not create something that was not there previously, it just enables people to use their unconscious capacities. Most of these hidden, unconscious capacities are utilized in one form or another in the normal course of events, but examples of their use are usually overlooked. For example, experiences of amnesia,

anesthesia, automatic movement, and even hallucinations occur very frequently, but in a manner that the conscious mind
ignores or accepts as ordinary without recognizing the reservoir of abilities that must underlie such occurrences. Hypnosis
merely brings these underlying abilities to the surface of
awareness and uses them directly.

The unconscious outstrips the conscious in all of its perceptual, conceptual, emotional, and response capabilities. It is or
contains everything that the conscious mind overlooks, ignores
or rejects *plus* everything that the conscious mind contains as
well. The unconscious has access to and can use almost everything that occurs or exists within the conscious mind but the
conscious mind generally is excluded from or protected from
the contents and potentials of the unconscious.

> **Most people do not know of their total capacities for
> response to stimuli. They place mystical meanings on
> much of the information they get by subtle cues.**
> *(Erickson, Rossi & Rossi, 1976, pp. 247-248)*

> **All of us have a tremendous number of generally
> unrecognized psychological and somatic learnings and
> conditionings. [circa 1950's]**
> *(In Erickson, 1980, Vol. IV, chap. 21, p. 224)*

> **The average person is unaware of the extent of his
> capacities of accomplishment which have been learned
> through the experiential conditionings of this body
> behavior through his life experiences. [1967]**
> *(In Erickson, 1980, Vol IV, chap. 24, p. 237)*

> **Every person has abilities not known to the self,
> abilities that can be expressed in trance.**
> **Memories, thoughts, feelings, sensations completely or
> partially forgotten by the conscious mind. Yet they are**

available to the unconscious and can be experienced within trance now or later whenever the unconscious is ready. [1976]

(In Erickson, 1980, Vol. I, chap. 22, p. 468)

The unconscious mind is made up of all your learnings over a lifetime, many of which you have completely forgotten, but which serve you in your automatic functioning. Now, a great deal of your behavior is the automatic functioning of these forgotten memories.

(Zeig, 1980, p. 33)

It's very charming, the capacity that we have if we'll only learn to use other areas of our brain.

(ASCH, 1980, Taped Lecture, 7/16/65)

When you stop and think about it, nobody does know his capacities.

(Erickson, Rossi & Rossi, 1976, p. 36)

Little is really known of the actual potentials of human functioning. [1970]

(In Erickson, 1980, Vol. IV, chap. 6, p. 53)

Every person has abilities not known to the self. [1976–78]

(In Erickson, 1980, Vol. I, chap. 22, p. 468)

Consciousness does not have available all the knowledge that is in the unconscious, which actually governs our perceptions and behavior.

(Erickson & Rossi, 1979, p. 367)

That patient may actually be governed by unconscious forces and emotions neither overtly shown nor even known. [1965]

(In Erickson, 1980, Vol. IV, chap. 20, p. 212)

> The problem yet remaining is to ensure that the
> members of the medical profession fully realize that the
> thinking, the emotions, and the past experiential learn-
> ings of each person can play a significant role in his
> psychological and physiological functionings. [1970]
>> *(In Erickson, 1980, Vol. IV, chap. 6, p. 58)*

The Unconscious is Brilliant

Given the above attributes of the unconscious in comparison
to the conscious mind, it is not surprising that Erickson
observed the unconscious to be "...much smarter, wiser and
quicker" than the conscious mind. It has access to more information than does the conscious mind and can analyze and
review that information without the biasing influences of
pride, prejudice, or expectation. In a sense, it represents the
innate intellectual potential of each individual were that individual to function at peak capacity.

It must be mentioned that in spite of its comparative
brilliance, the unconscious is not infallible. On occasion it can
and does arrive at erroneous or illogical conclusions. Also, it is
not surperhuman and is subject to normal physiological and
perceptual limitations. It cannot and does not know what it
has no reason to know on the basis of experience. Although it
may seem miraculous at times, it is not. It only seems so in
comparison to what we generally believe to be the normal
capacities and abilities of people.

> Now what people don't *know*...it's infinite...things
> that they actually do know but believe that they don't
> know.
>> *(Zeig, 1980, p. 179)*

> **We all have so much knowledge of which we are unaware.**
>
> *(Erickson, Rossi & Rossi, 1976, p.247)*

> **The unconscious mind is very brilliant.**
>
> *(Erickson & Rossi, 1979, p.312)*

> **The unconscious is much smarter, wiser, and quicker. It understands better.**
>
> *(Erickson & Rossi, 1979, p. 302)*

The Unconscious is Aware

One of the most significant and paradoxical aspects of the unconscious mind is that it is not unconscious at all. It is, on the contrary, extremely aware of and responsive to everything that occurs. It is unconscious only in the sense that the conscious mind is oblivious to its presence, to its ongoing operations, to its attempts to communicate, and to its influences upon ordinary thought, perception and behavior. Our awareness or unconsciousness of it gives it its name, not any lack of awareness on its part.

Erickson often noted that people are unconsciously aware of much more than they are consciously. Of particular significance is the ability of an individual to be much more aware unconsciously of the unconscious activities and responses of another person that either of them can be consciously. In an interaction between two people, the unconscious mind of each is busy being aware of the unconscious activities of the other while, in all probability, neither person is consciously aware of those activities. What this amounts to is an ongoing, surreptitious level of communication that may end up having as much influence on the interaction as the conscious level of communication. Obviously, anyone interested in being a therapist would do well to learn how to become aware of and to use this unconscious ability to decipher the unconscious communications of another. They should know what their own unconscious is communicating to the patient's unconscious as well. Such exchanges could have a significant impact on the progress of therapy and should be monitored carefully.

> **There also should be a ready and full respect for the patient's unconscious mind to perceive fully the intentionally obscured meaningful therapeutic instructions offered them. [1966]**
>
> *(In Erickson, 1980, Vol. IV, chap. 28, p. 277)*

> **One should also give recognition to the readiness with which one's unconscious mind picks up clues and information. [1966]**
>
> *(In Erickson, 1980, Vol. IV, chap. 28, p. 277)*

> **Because a person's unconscious mind tends to listen and tends to single out those things. Any six-months-old baby can look at mother's face as mother spoons some pablum toward the baby and read in great big headlines on mother's face "Who on Earth could stand the taste of that stuff?" And the baby agrees and spits it out.**
>
> *(ASCH, 1980, Taped Lecture, 2/2/66)*

> **Your unconscious mind understands very well and can work hard. [1964]**
>
> *(In Erickson, 1980, Vol. I, chap. 13, p. 323)*

> **Respectful awareness of the capacity of the patient's unconscious mind to perceive meaningfulness of the therapist's own unconscious behavior is a governing principle in psychotherapy. [1966]**
>
> *(In Erickson, 1980, Vol. IV, chap. 28, p. 277)*

The Unconscious Perceives and Responds Literally

Conceptual frameworks, perceptual categorizations, biases, judgements, and expectations are the province of the conscious mind. The unconscious level of awareness or mentation usually is characterized by the absence of these influences. As a consequence, the unconscious typically involves a more objective and less distorted awareness of reality than the conscious.

Erickson described the unconscious perception and knowledge of reality as direct, unbiased, and literal. The unconscious absorbs and knows about reality on the basis of simple, concrete experiences rather than on the basis of complex interpretations or explanations. It does not filter or distort material to suit its perspective or framework because it does not have one. It is not constrained by a specific context and can respond to events without the limitations imposed by contextually derived meanings. It simply perceives, processes, and reacts to whatever *is* in a direct or literal manner. Its perceptions, understandings, and responses are, therefore, more akin to those of a child who has yet to learn the rigid rules, judgements, biases, and filters of an adult. It does not "read meaning into" a statement or an event, but responds in a literal or multi-contextual manner. Normally, it does not impose contexts, although it may allow the event to determine the context or it may impose a context suggested to it by a hypnotist. All contexts or perspectives are available to it, although, generally, unconscious awareness is simple, direct, and literal, as are unconscious responses.

Paradoxically, the literal awareness that occurs at an unconscious level is probably responsible for the ability of the unconscious to understand and utilize complex metaphors, puns, analogies, and symbolism of all kinds in ways that may seem to be astoundingly creative to our restricted conscious intellects. It seems illogical that literalism would provide a creative outcome, but the relationship may be clarified by reiterating the point that to be literal means not to be constrained by or responsive to contextually implied meanings.

For example, when we hear the word "run," we normally determine what is meant by the context within which it occurs. The unconscious response to the word "run," however, is not contextually bound because it does not abide by or impose any particular perspective or cognitive contexts upon the word. The significance of this fact becomes more apparent when the following sentence is considered: "The watch runs." Everyone recognizes and tends to respond to the implied meaning of "run" in this statement but notice what happens if we allow ourselves to respond to it literally, i.e. without contextual restraints. We may, as a result, imagine a watch with legs running, a watch running like water out of a faucet, a watch running like the dye in cloth, etc. Any of these images is a possible literal interpretation; from a literal standpoint each is a legitimate visual representation of what was said. Even more creative expressions of this statement can occur is we free ourselves from the contextually implied meaning of "watch."

Erickson's recognition of the literalism of the unconscious evidently enabled him to communicate a literal message unconsciously via metaphors and puns while the patient responded consciously to the surface meaning of his statements. It also apparently enabled him to understand the so-called "symbolism" of dreams by reacting to their literal meanings, rather than to their contextual or implied meanings.

Finally, the literalism available at the unconscious level of awareness provides a source of objective, detached perception. Events or memories that might be impossible to consider because of their personal significance or their conflict with conscious beliefs, values, and attitudes becomes interesting and informative when viewed from within the objective perspective of the unconscious.

> **The unconscious is literal and tends to accept only what is said.**
>
> *(Erickson & Rossi, 1979, p. 431)*

> *R:* **The unconscious knows reality from concrete experiences.**
> *E:* **Yes.**
>
> *(Erickson, Rossi, & Rossi, 1976, p. 218)*

> **The secondary-level suggestion depends upon the literalism of the unconscious.**
>
> *(Erickson & Rossi, 1979, p. 162)*

> **He answered questions simply and briefly, giving literally and precisely no more and no less than the literal significance of the questions implied. [1965]**
>
> *(In Erickson, 1980, Vol. I, chap. 3, p. 94)*

The Unconscious is Childlike

It is not surprising that children are more in touch with or more able to utilize their unconscious minds than are adults. Their conscious minds have yet to dissociate completely as rigidly structured and separate systems of functioning so children necessarily continue to participate in and to utilize their unconscious levels of literal awareness and learning. As a result, the behavior and styles of children represent the basic character of an adult's unconscious. The unconscious is childlike.

Erickson remarked on several occasions that children are much more responsive to unconscious processes and are much more observant than adults. He also noted that they are more responsive to hypnosis, an observation that has been supported consistently by empirical research.

How many of us really appreciate the childishness of the unconscious mind? Because the unconscious mind is decidedly simple, unaffected, straightforward and honest. It hasn't got all of this facade, this veneer of what we call adult culture. It's rather simple, rather childish.
(ASCH, 1980, Taped Lecture, 2/2/66)

A parallel can be drawn between those infants who have not yet learned the realities of life and the putting aside of learned realities that can be observed as an entirely spontaneous manifestation in the hypnotic trance, most clearly so in the somnambulistic state. [1967]
(In Erickson, 1980, Vol. I, chap. 2, p. 76)

When you have a patient in a trance, the patient thinks like a child and reaches for an understanding.
(Erickson, Rossi & Rossi, 1976, p. 255)

The unconscious is much more childlike in that it is direct and it is free.
(Erickson, Rossi & Rossi, 1976, p. 255)

The Unconscious is the Source of Emotions

Emotions often burst forth into awareness unbidden, unwanted, and usually not understood. In general, emotions come from the unconscious. As psychophysiological expressions they typically are reflections of unconscious feelings about or reactions to the situation, usually as that situation relates to the conscious personality. Emotions are not logical, rational, or conscious, but they are a natural and potentially useful form of unconscious communication. They tell us how we feel about something even when we are unaware of how we feel.

> *R:* **Feelings come from our unconscious.**
> *E:* **Yes.**
> *(Erickson, Rossi & Rossi, 1976, p. 182)*

> **Emotional reactions are not necessarily rational, especially so at an unconscious level of reaction. [1952]**
> *(In Erickson, 1980, Vol. I, chap. 6, p. 151)*

> **Explosiveness is a sudden welling up of the unconscious and everyone has had that experience.**
> *(Erickson & Rossi, 1979, p. 227)*

The Unconscious is Universal

Erickson reached the conclusion that the unconscious is a fairly uniform, similar set of processes from one individual to another on the basis of his observations of multiple personalities, hypnotized subjects and the similarities of rituals and beliefs across cultural and historical contexts. He was, for example, much impressed by the similarities of the drawings of psychotics from different cultures and different centuries.

Even though tentative and not easily observable, the universality of the unconscious, its similarity from one person to another, formed an important aspect of his general understanding of people. The unconscious, it would appear, knows no national, cultural, or historical boundaries; it speaks in a literal manner and uses a form of thought that understands the unconscious of another much more effectively than could the conscious mind of either person. Obviously, the more similar the life experiences of any two people are, the more true this is, but any two people growing up in this world would have enough similar experiences to make it more true than not.

The unconscious seems to reflect the fact that all people are, originally, just plain human beings with essentially identical neurophysiological capacities and an innate tendency to learn, to respond, and to perceive in particular ways. In many respects, most of Erickson's comments regarding the unconscious might be considered to be descriptions of the basic nature of, the innate capacities of, and the response tendencies of human beings in general. His description of the unconscious seems to be a description of a fundamental aspect of people; a description that is neither psychoanalytic, nor humanistic, nor behavioral but is simply an objective description of what all people are, do, and are capable of doing originally and continuously beneath the level of their divergent conscious frames of reference.

There must be individual differences in the contents of the unconscious because every unconscious contains only the information or impressions provided by the unique experiential learning history of the particular unique individual. But the fundamental form, structure, or pattern of response of every human unconscious may be very similar indeed. It would appear that people are both fundamentally different and fundamentally similar.

> **Your unconscious behaves in accord with its own code of behavior.**
>
> *(ASCH, 1980, Taped Lecture, 2/2/66)*

Human thinking and human emotion the world over through all of our records is very much the same, that we can all get the same ideas in various disordered states.

(ASCH, 1980, Taped Lecture, 8/14/66)

Underneath the diversified nature of the consciously organized aspects of the personality, the unconscious talks in a language which has a remarkable uniformity; further, that that language has laws so constant that the unconscious of one individual is better equipped to understand the unconscious of another than the conscious aspects of the personality of either. [1938]

(In Erickson, 1980, Vol. III, chap. 19, p. 186)

The similarities [between various pictures and dreams] were amazing, until one realizes that the dreams and the pictures come from essentially similar minds even though from different mental states and cultures. [1964]

(In Erickson, 1980, Vol. I, chap. 14, p. 338)

Thus, the common dream symbolism of the mentally ill patients of India and the United States; the common symbolism in the art work of the mentally ill German patients of an earlier era and those of newly admitted mentally ill patients in the United States; the translation of cryptic automatic writing of one hypnotic subject by another subject; along with this report on the Pantomime Technique in hypnosis, all suggest the following: That a parallelism of thought and comprehension processes exists which is not based upon verbalizations evocative of specified responses, but which derives from behavioral manifestations not ordinarily recognized or appreciated at the conscious level of mentation. [1964]

(In Erickson, 1980, Vol. I, chap. 14, p.338)

> **In other words, this boy was simply a human being,
> with a human mind competent and capable of working
> along the patterns that the human mind is capable of
> working. And it was utterly amazing the way this boy's
> productions could be paralleled.**
>
> *(ASCH, 1980, Taped Lecture, 8/14/66)*

Summary

Erickson's observations led him to the conclusion that people actually have an unconscious mind that is separate from conscious awareness. This unconscious mind perceives, thinks and responds to the world in a literal or objective fashion unimpaired by the rigidities and biases of the conscious mind. It sees things the conscious mind ignores, it knows things the conscious mind overlooks, and it remembers things the conscious mind has forgotten. It takes responsibility for many complex activities such as walking, driving a car, reading, etc. It often influences the thoughts, perceptions, and behavior of the conscious mind by providing "intuitive" hunches, educated guesses, dream experiences, and emotional responses. Although childlike in many respects, it actually is wiser and more perceptive than the conscious mind. It contains a vast range of unrecognized capabilities and potentials, some of which are used in an unnoticed fashion on a daily basis. Many of these capabilities, however, lie dormant and unused because of the restraints and concerns of the conscious mind.

Finally, the unconscious is a universal attribute. No matter how different people are in their conscious realms of existence, they remain linked by the qualities and capacities of their unconscious minds. Diverse cultural backgrounds do not seem to prevent clear communication and understanding at the unconscious level of awareness.

CHAPTER FOUR

NORMALCY AND PATHOLOGY

It should be apparent from the descriptions presented in the previous chapters that Erickson did not view people as inherently or typically perfect. On the contrary, the normal development of the conscious mind and the general inability to use many of the processes and capabilities of the unconscious mind would seem destined to produce a population of rather imperfect, illogical, prejudiced, and even downright strange individuals. Indeed, this appears to be exactly what Erickson saw as he looked about him. Rather than becoming depressed or upset about the universal imperfection of people, however, he accepted and embraced it as a desirable quality. He even warned therapists not to strive for or demand perfection in their patients, but to accept and utilize the unique and often bizarre qualities that they presented.

If imperfection is an acceptable and normal trait, then we may well wonder exactly what therapists should strive to cure.

What aspects of human behavior are undesirable or abnormal and in need of improvement or change? The material in this chapter provides Erickson's answer to that question. The quotations reviewed below define the nature and source of psychopathological phenomena, thereby setting the stage for an understanding of his goals and strategies of psychotherapy. This material derives directly from his basic orientation toward life, that people should observe and use what *is* in order to meet their needs, attain their goals or accomplish their purposes, and relies upon his observations regarding conscious and unconscious functioning. As a result, what is presented here is not really new but, like much of the material in the remainder of this book, is merely a natural extension of his more fundamental observations. It is, nevertheless, of paramount importance to the development of an overall comprehension of an Ericksonian approach to hypnosis and psychotherapy.

What is Abnormal?

Abnormality was a relative term for Erickson. He maintained that the same behavior could be viewed as abnormal in one situation but as normal in another. The temper tantrum of one child could be an intelligent and adaptive response, while the purposeless temper tantrum of another might be a sign of abnormality. Similarly, the various phenomena of hypnosis are desirable abilities when manifested under the direction of a hypnotist but are potentially unproductive pathological occurrences under uncontrolled circumstances.

The differentiating features of abnormal and normal behavior were specified clearly by Erickson. *Any behavior that does not serve a useful and meaningful goal for the person, that is at variance with that individual's personality, or that actually interferes with that person's ability to attain reasonable personal goals is abnormal or undesirable.* This emphasis upon the nonutilitarian features of abnormal behavior appears to be a natural extension of his basic orientation toward life and it gives a special flavor to his hypnotherapeutic approach. Interestingly enough, however, it is a view that he rarely expressed in a direct manner and, consequently, all but one of the following quotes were taken from the same source.

> And so, when recognition is given to the fact that everyone is queer in some respects, the question arises, "By what means, criterion or yardstick may judgement of abnormality be passed effectively and correctly?"
>
> *(Erickson, 1941a, p. 100)*

> Abnormal behavior, on the other hand, is not purposeful in a clearly understandable, recognizable, and effective fashion, and it is primarily directed to goals that are not in keeping or harmony with what one properly expects of that individual.
>
> *(Erickson, 1941a, p. 101)*

> However, this does not necessarily mean that the purpose and goal of human behavior must necessarily be legitimate and desirable, since human nature is not perfect. Normal human behavior can be subject to prejudices, misunderstandings, ignorance, and to all the weaknesses of mankind, and yet have purposes and goals readily understood and appreciated as being harmonious to an individual possessed of normal desires and strivings, regardless of any errors of judgement and the lack of common sense in his behavior.
>
> *(Erickson, 1941a, p. 101)*

Thus, behavior that does not serve a readily understandable and useful goal for the individual, that is not in keeping with what may reasonably be expected of that person, that is persisted in to such an extent that it interferes with the person's other and understandably useful behavior, is definitely abnormal.

(Erickson, 1941a, p. 101)

In other words, to be abnormal, behavior must necessarily be lacking in purposeful useful qualities so far as the reasonably average goals of the specific individual person are concerned.

(Erickson, 1941a, p. 101)

The general practitioner needs primarily to judge his patient's behavior in terms of what may reasonably be expected of that particular individual, in terms of what is purposeful and useful to the individual and in terms of what behavior is in keeping and harmony with the general established patterns of behavior of the specific person.

(Erickson, 1941 a, p. 108)

As one views the schizophrenic patient and looks over his life history, one is impressed repeatedly by the lack of understandable purposefulness in his behavior, the uselessness of many things that he does and the general tendency toward infantile and childish behavior, which would be suggestive in a small child of a behavior disorder.

(Erickson, 1941a, p. 107)

On the basis of my knowledge of psychiatry, psychotic behavior is disturbed, uncontrolled, and misdirected behavior which the individual has limited ability to change, modify, or understand. ...In psychosis there is

the wrong behavior, in the wrong place, usually at the
wrong time. [1960]

(In Erickson, 1980, Vol. II, chap. 31, p. 326)

The neurotic's complaints, however unreal physically,
do dominate, limit and restrict normal functioning as
much as does actual physical disease.

(Erickson, 1941a, p. 106)

These symptoms are real to the patient, and when they
interfere seriously with that person's social, economic
and personal adjustments, when they cause his behavior
to become purposeless and useless, adequate recognition
and attention should be given to these complaints.

(Erickson, 1941a, p. 106)

Conscious Sources of Abnormality

Although Erickson rarely provided direct statements of his
definition of abnormality, he did allude to it whenever he
discussed the pathological consequences of conscious attitudes
or mental sets. Conscious sets or biases were viewed as the
typical source of difficulties or abnormalities in learning and
performance by Erickson. The behavior of the conscious mind
often leads to bias, confusion, and even interference with unconscious capacities and can result in a disruption of performance, an inability to profit from experience and an inability
to attain one's goals. Abnormality, therefore, often stems
directly from the interfering, inept and non-objective activities
of the conscious mind which too often strives for understandings, even erroneous or limiting understandings, at the expense
of a general awareness of experiences and an unconscious
"feeling" for how best to conduct oneself.

As an aside, it may be worth noting that the comments contained in the following section probably could be used to explain the lack of specificity of Erickson's various presentations. They suggest that Erickson was concerned that others develop a "feeling" for or "sense" of his perspective rather than a conceptual explanation or understanding of it or of his techniques.

In the ordinary state of conscious awareness performance is too often limited by considerations which may actually be unrelated to the task. [1970]
(In Erickson, 1980, Vol. IV, chap. 6, p. 55)

Ideas, understandings, beliefs, wishes, hopes, and fears can all impinge easily upon a performance in the state of ordinary awareness — disrupting and distorting even those goals which may have been singly desired. [1970]
(In Erickson, 1980, Vol. IV, chap. 6, p. 55)

Their failure in the waking state resulted not from incapacity, since capacity had been demonstrated, but from a mental set, contingent upon wakefulness, precluding the initiation of the remote preliminary mental processes leading to the actual performance. [1938]
(In Erickson, 1980, Vol. II, chap. 10 p. 99)

The blinding effects of emotional bias. [1948]
(In Erickson, 1980, IV, chap. 4, p. 44)

Don't let conscious frames of reference occlude your vision.
(Erickson, Rossi & Rossi, 1976, p. 209)

People assume so much.
(Zeig, 1980, p. 354)

You are letting your intellect interfere with your learning.

(Zeig, 1980, p. 42)

The conscious mind understands the logic of it, and the unconscious understands the reality.

(Erickson, Rossi & Rossi, 1967, p. 218)

Confusion results from trying to impose some form of regimentation upon natural processes.

(Erickson, Rossi & Rossi, 1976, p. 243)

R: That rational approach is good for certain intellectual things, but for total human functioning it is not good.
E: It's *not* good!

(Erickson, Rossi & Rossi, 1976, p. 251)

It would spoil the magician's art if you knew how he did that trick. If you want to enjoy swimming, do not analyze it. If you want to make love, don't try to analyze it.

(Erickson, Rossi & Rossi, 1976, p. 255)

The feeling is the essential thing. Knowing about it is not the essential thing.

(Erickson & Rossi, 1976, p. 164)

The best way of learning, to use folk language, is by getting the feel of it. You get the feel of a poem, the feeling of a picture, the feeling of a statue. Feeling is a very meaningful word. We do not just feel with the fingers, but with the heart, the mind. You feel with the learnings of the past. You feel with the hopes for the future. You feel the present.

(Erickson, Rossi & Rossi, 1976, p. 253)

> **Too often the conscious behavior keeps you too busy so you deprive the unconscious of an opportunity to express itself. It's another scientific truism.**
>
> *(Erickson, Rossi & Rossi, 1976, p. 38)*

> **This illustrates the biasing influence of a conscious set on true knowledge.**
>
> *(Erickson, Rossi & Rossi, 1976, p. 209)*

Rigidity of Abnormality

Given that much of the abnormality confronting a psychotherapist is the manifestation or consequence of certain conscious biases or sets, the obvious solution would be to alter or eliminate those biases and sets. This sounds easy but every experienced therapist knows that it is not. The conscious mind evolves into a very rigid structure, one that resists experiencing things that cause it to change. The earlier a pathology-inducing attitude was absorbed into that structure the more resistant it seems to be to change and the more likely the individual is to persist in the abnormal behavior. Any attempt to argue somebody out of a deeply ingrained conscious mental set that probably was initiated and supported by the family or the culture usually will prove to be a futile endeavor. If anything, such attempts will initiate frantic efforts to further defend the pathology-inducing ideation.

> **When we were very young, we were willing to learn. And the older we grow, the more restrictions we put on ourselves.**
>
> *(Zeig, 1980, p. 75)*

And for human behavior — we start from childhood to become rigid, very rigid in our behavior, only we don't know that. We think that we are being free, but we are not. And we ought to recognize it.

(Zeig, 1980, p. 117)

Those early maladjustments serve to establish and to fix within the individual unhealthy and abnormal ways of behaving so that the individual becomes progressively more handicapped in his general life situation.

(Erickson, 1941a, p. 102)

Those deviations from the normal in children do lead to a greater susceptibility to mental illness.

(Erickson, 1941a, p. 104)

Their complaints constitute essentially the childhood behavior disorders grown older and larger.

(Erickson, 1941a, p. 106)

The reader should bear in mind that the hold of social conventions upon the patients also played a significant role in both their illness and their therapy.

(Erickson, 1980, Vol. IV, p. xxii)

And people are so very, very rigid. And each ethnic group has its do's and don'ts.

(Zeig, 1980, p. 120)

We have billions of brain cells that have the capacity to respond to billions of different stimuli, and the brain cells are very specialized. When you come from people who generation after generation only use certain brain cells, every signal that you get as an infant centers you around that.. ...You see, while we're born with similar brain cells, there's a pattern of response that's inherent in our behavior.. ...Ingrained so that you indirectly warn the child away from their natural response.

(Zeig, 1980, p. 340)

The tendency for one pattern of thinking to persist, and the difficulty in shifting to another type, are generally recognized. [1937]

(In Erickson, 1980, Vol. III, chap. 16, p. 149)

I discussed in general the fixity of the subject's beliefs and the general imperviousness to any reasoning approach to her delusional ideas. A parallel was drawn between this behavior and the general attitude taken by the psychotic patient when a reasoning approach is made to any form of abnormal ideation. [1939]

(In Erickson, 1980, Vol. III, chap. 20, p. 205)

When you understand how man really defends his intellectual ideas and how emotional he gets about it, you should realize that the first thing in psychotherapy is not to try to compel him to change his ideation; rather you go along with it and change it in a gradual fashion and create situations wherein he himself willingly changes his thinking. [1977]

(In Erickson, 1980, Vol. IV, chap. 36, p. 335)

The Protection of Abnormality

Part of the problem with direct frontal assaults upon the pathology-inducing ideation of the conscious mind is that the ideation and structure of the conscious mind are thoroughly protected. Even before patients enter the therapist's office, they will probably have constructed a rather massive system of conscious and unconscious protections for the particular pattern of thought that supports or initiates their pathological symptoms. In fact, many of the symptoms presented by patients actually are devices constructed or used by them to protect the structure of their conscious minds from potentially profitable but threatening experiences and understandings.

The unconscious automatically protects the conscious mind when conscious vulnerabilities make it necessary to do so, even to the point of preventing the conscious from becoming unpleasantly aware of the ideas or behaviors underlying emotional problems. Patients, therefore, are people who have been unwilling or unable to view themselves, others or their situation objectively and who even may have unconsciously constructed a more or less elaborate set of protective responses that will enable them to continue in their distorted and ineffectual awareness of reality.

> **Those personality traits disliked by the self are easily repressed from conscious awareness and are rapidly recognized in others or projected upon others. [1948]**
> *(In Erickson, 1980, vol. IV, chap. 4, p. 43)*

> **The conscious mind already has its own set ideas about the neurosis. It has its fixed, rigid perceptions that constitute a neurotic set. It's very difficult to get people at the conscious level to accept an alteration of their general thinking about themselves. [1973]**
> *(In Erickson, 1980 Vol. III, chap. 11, p. 100)*

> **The neurotic is self-protective of the neurosis. [1973]**
> *(In Erickson, 1980, Vol. III, chap. 11, p. 100)*

> **Man is characterized not only by mobility but by cognition and by emotion, and man defends his intellect emotionally. [1977]**
> *(In Erickson, 1980, Vol. IV, chap. 36, p. 335)*

No two people necessarily have the same ideas, but all people will defend their ideas whether they are psychotically based or culturally based, or nationally based or personally based. [1977]
(In Erickson, 1980, Vol. III, chap. 36, p. 335)

The development of neurotic symptoms constitutes behavior of a defensive protective character. Because it is an unconscious process, excluded from conscious understandings, it is blind and groping in nature, does not serve personality purposes usefully, and tends to be handicapping and disabling in its effects.
(Erickson, 1954d, p. 109)

Unconscious conflict and indecision within the psyche gives rise to anxiety against which defenses are erected. [1944]
(In Erickson, 1980, Vol. III, chap. 21, p. 216)

The unconscious always protects the conscious.
(Erickson, Rossi & Rossi, 1976, p. 13)

R: Does the unconscious *always* protect the person?
E: Yes, but often in ways that the conscious mind does not understand.
(Erickson & Rossi, 1979, p. 296)

Unconsciously you don't have to do what you consciously say you will. In everyday life, you may accept an invitation for dinner, and later your unconscious lets you forget it.
(Erickson & Rossi, 1979, p. 315)

Good unconscious understandings allowed to become conscious before a conscious readiness exists will result in conscious resistance, rejection, repression and even the loss, through repression, of unconscious gains. [1948]
(In Erickson,, 1980, Vol. IV, chap. 4, p. 41)

The unconscious is going to be protective of consciousness. It is going to try to reassure the conscious mind with "You don't have to be depressed if you didn't do things." The unconscious won't say "You did something even though you didn't know it." It doesn't function that way. It just says "You don't have to worry because you failed."
(Erickson, Rossi & Rossi, 1976, p. 208)

Utilizing the patient's own neurotic irrationality to affirm and confirm a simple extension of his neurotic fixation relieved him of all unrecognized unconscious needs to defend his neuroticism against all assaults. [1965]
(In Erickson 1980, Vol. IV, chap. 20, p. 218)

A remarkable illustration of the intensity and effectiveness with which the body can provide defenses for psychological reasons. [1954]
(In Erickson, 1980, Vol. IV, chap. 14, p. 170)

By this utterance the patient demonstrated the protectiveness of the unconscious for the conscious. [1948]
(In Erickson, 1980, Vol. IV, chap. 4, p. 40)

Your unconscious mind knows what is right and what is good. When you need protection, it will protect you.
(Erickson & Rossi, 1979, p. 296)

You have all the protection of your own unconscious, which has been protecting you in your dreams, permitting you to dream what you wish, when you wish, and keeping that dream as long as your unconscious thought necessary, or as long as your conscious mind thought would be desirable.

(Erickson, Rossi & Rossi, 1976, p. 35)

And your unconscious mind can keep from you, from your conscious mind, anything it doesn't want you to know consciously.

(Erickson & Lustig, 1975, Vol. 1, p. 9)

You don't know just how much your unconscious wants you to know.

(Erickson & Rossi, 1977, p. 50)

These defenses prevent both unconscious resolution of the conflict and its emergence into consciousness, and may result in inhibition of thinking, confusion, interference with activity. [1944]

(In Erickson, 1980, Vol. III, chap. 21, p. 216)

The conscious mind downgrades unconscious accomplishments, and you can't allow that downgrading to continue because conscious emotions filter down to the unconscious.

(Erickson, Rossi & Rossi, 1976, p. 208)

Yes, it [conscious] can limit itself. The things I say are consciously heard but are understood on an unconscious level only. But the unconscious can keep those sexual connotations to itself. You don't allow the self to become aware of it.

(Erickson & Rossi, 1979, p. 154)

We all realize that personality reactions and emotional attitudes may manifest themselves directly or indirectly, consciously or at a level at which people are unaware of their conduct, or if they become aware of their conduct, may be unaware of their motivations. **[1939]**
(In Erickson, 1980, Vol. IV, chap. 1, p. 12)

"A patient himself is a person who is afraid to be direct."
(In Beahrs, 1977, p. 57)

Forms of Abnormality

Pathological symptoms and complaints are either expressions of a faulty underlying conscious set or the results of mechanisms used to defend the person against the recognition of something unpleasant. Erickson often employed the Freudian classifications of such defense mechanisms and seemed to be especially intrigued by the processes of repression and dissociation. He postulated that all acts of repression may generate new and separate personalities, a postulate that may further explain the development of the conscious and unconscious minds. In many respects, the conscious/unconscious dichotomy seems to be a dissociation created by repression. Consequently, it is not unreasonable to conclude that Erickson's observations indicated that everyone is a dual personality. The typical separation between the conscious and the unconscious minds seems to be comparable in source and effect to the division that occurs in multiple personalities.

The dissociative process also was of interest to Erickson because he found that it could be a valuable circumstance in the hypnotherapeutic process. He actually used the hypnotic trance to enhance the conscious/unconscious dissociation of a patient so that he could communicate directly with the unconscious mind while the conscious awareness was focused elsewhere.

Be that as it may, the following comments are offered as an expression of his perception of various psychopathological conditions and symptoms, including multiple personalities.

I don't know what the mechanism of displacement is, but I do know that human beings make use of that mechanism. [1960]

(In Erickson, 1980, Vol. II, chap. 31, p. 317)

However, the history of psychopathology is replete with evidence to show that the human mind, however lacking it may be in fundamental endowments, needs little instruction in devising complex escape mechanisms. [1932]

(In Erickson, 1980, Vol. I, chap. 24, p. 497)

Against this, she originally defended herself by a partial dissociation and an attempted identification with her grandfather. [1939]

(In Erickson, 1980, Vol. III, chap. 23, p. 258)

Clearly, in the production of the multiple personality, a process must occur in which certain psychological events are rendered unconscious. [1939]

(In Erickson, 1980, Vol. III, chap. 23, p. 256)

In fact, one must ask whether one is justified in dismissing the possibility that all acts of repression involve the creation of a larval form of a secondary personality. [1939]

(In Erickson, 1980, Vol. III, chap. 23, pp. 256–257)

The "repression" which would result in a multiple personality would be a vertical division of one personality into two more or less complete units like the splitting of a paramecium. [1939]

(In Erickson, 1980, Vol. III, chap. 23, p. 256)

The states of conscious and unconscious mentation existing in cases of multiple personality *coexist* quite as truly as in simpler repressions. [1939]

(In Erickson, 1980, Vol. III, chap. 23, p. 257)

The person with dual or multiple personalities must necessarily have constructed them out of a single experiential background. Hence, any differences in the personalities constructed must reflect differing uses, differing qualities of activeness or passiveness for the same items in this experiential background. [circa 1940's]

(In Erickson, 1980, Vol. III, chap. 24, p. 267)

Hence, I would stress as an adequate measure of discovery for multiple personalities any procedure of systematic clinical observation that would permit the recognition of different sets and patterns of behavior integration and a determination of the interrelationships between various organizations of behavior reactions. [circa 1940's]

(In Erickson, 1980, Vol. III, chap. 24, p. 263)

Inevitably, this raises the question of how frequent such unrecognized dual personalities may be, either as partial or complete formations. [1939]

(In Erickson, 1980, Vol. III, chap. 23, p. 255)

It is possible also that the unsuspected presence of just such dual personalities, closely knit and completely segregated from the rest of the personality, may account for certain analytic defeats. [1939]
(In Erickson, 1980, Vol. III, chap. 23, p. 252)

Not infrequently in neurotic difficulties, there is a surrender of the personality to an overwhelming symptom-complex formation, which may actually be out of proportion to the maladjustment problem.
(Erickson, 1954d, pp.116–117)

Psychopathological manifestations need not necessarily be considered expressive of combined or multiple disturbances of several different modalities of behavior. Rather, they disclose that a disturbance in one single modality may actually be expressed in several other spheres of behavior as apparently unrelated coincidental disturbances. Hence, seemingly different symptoms may be but various aspects of a single manifestation for which the modalities of expression may properly be disregarded. [1943]
(In Erickson, 1980, Vol. II, chap. 14, p. 156)

Recovery from one illness (or conflict) frequently results in the establishment of a new physiological equilibrium (or "resolution of libido") thereby permitting the favorable resolution of a second concurrent and perhaps totally unrelated illness (or conflict).
An intercurrent disease may exercise a favorable effect upon the original illness, for example, malaria in paresis. [1935]
(In Erickson, 1980, Vol. III, chap. 28, p. 320)

The psychotherapeutic approach and the hypnotic approach [to stuttering], in my experience, are most effec-

> tive if you recognize one general factor. Stuttering is a
> form of aggression against society, and people in general.
>
> *(Erickson, 1977b, p. 32)*

> The extreme obsessional character of their behavior,
> thought, and emotions was most marked. They seemed,
> as persons, to be sound, yet caught in a situation they
> could not handle.
>
> *(Erickson & Rossi, 1979, p. 362)*

Minimizing Abnormality

It seems appropriate to conclude this brief chapter on abnormality and this introductory section on the general nature of people with some words about the ideal form of human functioning from Erickson's point of view. The following collection of quotations offers a straightforward and optimistic summary of his prescriptions for ideal, albeit imperfect functioning. The essence of his message seems to be that if people were able to confront and experience the realities of life openly and objectively and were able to accept and to use these experiences and the full range of their conscious and unconscious capacities, then generally they would be able to learn how to do the right thing, in the right way at the right time as defined by their unique goals and circumstances. They could overcome a majority of life's obstacles and problems and could live a creative, comfortable, and joyful existence full of wonderment at the unfolding of their own capacities.

Erickson's comments on the human potential to overcome adversities and to learn from them provides an effective backdrop for the subsequent presentation of his goals and strategies of psychotherapy in the next section of this book because many of the statements quoted here actually are the comments and suggestions he offered to his patients during hypnotherapy. They were not uttered as mere speculations on how nice life could be but were presented to open up new ways for his patients to think, act, and feel. They represent his goals for his patients and his prescription for effective living.

> **Among our patients here we can demonstrate many who were such model children that they never learned the realities of life. In other words, the diet of social development and health must include a reasonable amount of "roughage."**
>
> *(Erickson, 1941a, p 104)*

> **The Erickson family, in large part, looks upon illness and misfortune as part of the roughage of life.**
>
> *(Zeig, 1980, p. 185)*

> **Life is much better if sometimes it rains and sometimes it doesn't.**
>
> *(Erickson & Rossi, 1979, p. 266)*

> **"Erickson, you better face life as it really is.... You better face it, Erickson. All your life, you are going to be confronted with the unfairness of life."**
>
> *(Zeig, 1980, p. 210)*

> **I had to learn to reconcile myself to the unfairness of life.**
>
> *(Erickson & Rossi, 1977, p. 42)*

> **There are plenty of alternatives in any situation.... When you attend a session of group therapy, what on earth are you going to see? That is what you go there for.**
>
> *(Erickson & Rossi, 1981, p. 206)*

In other words, reacting to the good and the bad, and dealing with it adequately — that's the real joy in life.

(Erickson & Lustig, 1975, Vol. 2, p. 7)

Too many of us have the attitude, "It can happen to you but it can't happen to me." [Deleted name] took the attitude, "If it can happen to someone else it can happen to me," which is a very nice, intelligent attitude.

(ASCH, 1980, Taped Lecture, 8/8/64)

Because we all start dying when we are born. Some of us are faster than others. Why not live and enjoy, because you can wake up dead. You won't know about it. But somebody else will worry then. Until that time — enjoy life.

(Zeig, 1980, p. 269)

Life isn't something you can give an answer to today. You should enjoy the process of waiting, the process of becoming what you are. There is nothing more delightful than planting flower seeds and not knowing what kind of flowers are going to come up.

(Erickson & Rossi, 1979, p. 389)

Yes, you encourage patients to do all those simple little things that are their own right as growing creatures. You see, we don't know what our goals are. We learn our goals only in the process of getting there. "I don't know what I'm building but I'm going to enjoy building it and when I get through building it I'll know what it is." In doing psychotherapy you impress this upon patients. You don't know what a baby is going to become. Therefore, you take good care of it until it becomes what it will.

(Erickson & Rossi, 1979, p. 389)

What I want you to do is to begin being yourself. Accepting yourself. And knowing that you can control yourself. You want to do something. You control yourself. You focus your efforts. And it is a wonderful thing to explore, to discover the self.

(Erickson & Rossi, 1979, p. 387)

And we should be willing to feel, fully, the pleasures and the happiness that we want, as all our feelings are done by ourselves.

(Erickson & Lustig, 1975, Vol. 2, p. 6)

Everybody is like his fingerprints. They're one of a kind. And never will be another like you. And you need to enjoy, always being you. And you can't change it — just as fingerprints can't be changed.

(Erickson & Lustig, Vol. 1, p. 7)

The important thing always is to do the right thing at the right time. To know that you can rely on yourself. To let your unconscious feed to you the right information that permits you to do the right thing at the right time.

(Erickson, Rossi & Rossi, 1976, p. 260)

People who accomplish a great many things are people who have freed themselves from biases. These are the creative people.

(Erickson, Rossi & Rossi, 1976, p. 179)

The ideal person would be one who had a readiness to accept the interchange between the conscious and unconscious. Children are uncluttered by rigid conscious sets, and therefore children can see things that adults cannot.

(Erickson, Rossi & Rossi, 1976, p. 258)

Juvenility is far superior to senility.

(Erickson, Rossi & Rossi, 1976, p. 256)

There is nothing wrong with having rigid sets. But if you want to alter yourself in some way, you must be unashamedly aware that you do have sets and it's better to have a greater variety of sets.

(Erickson, Rossi & Rossi, 1976, p. 213)

It's a nice thing to learn because it will teach you objectivity which will enable you to do right things at the right time in the right way.

(Erickson, Rossi & Rossi, 1976, p. 158)

Summary

Erickson defined abnormal behavior as any behavior that did not serve a useful purpose for the individual. Furthermore, he concluded that abnormality usually is a consequence of rigid, highly protected, non-objective conscious mental sets which resist experiential learning. Normal behavior is productive and appropriate for the individual involved, although it need not be totally unprejudiced or reasonable because people are not inherently perfect. On the other hand, people do have the capacity to function very creatively, competently, and joyfully if they can overcome the self-limiting and destructive components of their rigid mental sets.

PSYCHOTHERAPY

PSYCHOTHERAPY

It should come as no surprise to learn that the goals, attitudes, and interventions used by Erickson in psychotherapy were derived from his observations on the basic nature of people and from his firm belief that effective living requires awareness, acceptance, and responsivity to the objective realities of life. What may come as a surprise is the depressing realization that one cannot become an Ericksonian psychotherapist simply by learning a specific set of Ericksonian therapy techniques.

In a very real sense, Ericksonian psychotherapy cannot be defined as a specific set of techniques nor can a therapist become an Ericksonian simply by memorizing and applying a particular group of techniques to patients. Erickson's underlying orientation and wisdom formed the well-spring from which his words and behaviors emerged. His techniques were tailored by his past and present observations to fit the peculiar demands of each moment; they were not firmly fixed or stylized routines.

What Erickson did in therapy was derived from his underlying framework and is definable as Ericksonian only because of this fact. Similarly, whatever is done by any therapist who has a similar orientation could be categorized as Ericksonian and, more importantly, any therapist who adopts an Ericksonian perspective probably will tend to engage in Ericksonian therapy automatically. Becoming an Ericksonian psychotherapist does not necessarily mean learning to *do* what Erickson did, but it does mean learning to think like Erickson thought. It means adopting an Ericksonian attitude toward people, toward therapy, and toward oneself as a therapist. It means developing an appreciation for the implications of an Ericksonian perspective and then accumulating the experientially and observationally based resources necessary to act upon those implications.

Obviously, the techniques used by a novice who only recently has developed an Ericksonian perspective will not be particularly unique or effective because that individual will not yet have acquired the requisite background of observations and experiences from which to respond effectively. The Ericksonian orientation provides the goals and attitudes, but not the means to the desired ends. Knowing what to do is not the same as knowing how to do it. For this reason, the observations, verbal and nonverbal skills, and general instructions provided by Dr. Erickson over the years may be useful tools for neophyte Ericksonians until they develop the observational and experiential basis for doing the right thing at the right time in their own way. The essential ingredients in becoming an Ericksonian, however, are the comprehension and incorporation of an Ericksonian orientation. Erickson stressed this point on numerous occasions and, accordingly, the material provided in the following chapters emphasizes the development of an overall, universally applicable sense or flavor of his approach rather than an accumulation of linguistically, culturally, or individually bound techniques. This material does not tell therapists exactly what to do in therapy, but it does tell them how to think so that they will know or be able to learn what to do. Such a teaching approach may demand a greater tolerance for ambiguity than the presentation of specifics and may require a greater dedication to conceptual and behavioral flexibility than the presentation of any answers. However, as the old saying goes, you can give a person a fish and feed him for a day or you can teach him how to fish and feed him for a lifetime. Erickson preferred to do the latter.

CHAPTER FIVE

THE GOAL OF PSYCHOTHERAPY

What happens during a therapy session is dependent to a large extent upon the goals and purposes of the therapist. The questions asked, the responses given, and the strategies used invariably are reflections of the underlying purpose of the psychotherapist. In fact, one of the major sources of differentiation between the various "schools" of therapy is the different goals that they have established for the patient and, by implication, for the therapist. Some strategies are designed to promote insight, others to maximize self-actualization, some to facilitate integration, and others simply to change inappropriate or undesirable responses. Whatever the goal, a great deal of the therapist's behavior is determined by it.

Erickson's goal for the therapeutic process was to facilitate the change to a new, preferably objective, perspective upon the presenting problem which would enable the person to use his or her own experientially acquired learnings in order to emit a more adaptive response to the situation. He often ignored insight and generally avoided perfectionism. Objective perception of an effective response to life's current situations was what he expected of himself and it was what he believed his patients required as well. The material presented below emphasizes these points and provides additional details regarding the general purposes of the Ericksonian psychotherapy process.

Focus on the Possible, Not on Perfection

Erickson did not expect his patients to be more than they were. He realized that nobody is perfect and that human faults are necessary and even desirable. His goal in therapy was not to create a perfect human being, but to help people learn how best to use their existing abilities and potentials, limited or faulty as they might be. By recognizing and accepting his patients' handicaps, he maintained an atmosphere of acceptance, protection, and trust and provided patients with attainable goals.

> **I object very seriously to this attitude of perfection that some physicians and dentists and psychologists have when dealing with human beings. I've never met a perfect human being yet and I never expect to meet one. I think the faults that you recall in human beings give their charm to that individual that enable you to recognize and remember that individual.**
>
> *(ASCH, 1980 Taped Lecture, 7/18/65)*

Long experience in psychotherapy has disclosed the wisdom of avoiding perfectionistic drives and wishes on the part of patients and of motivating them for the comfortable achievement of lesser goals. This then ensures not only the lesser goal but makes more possible the easy output of effort that can lead to a greater goal. Of even more importance is that the greater accomplishment then becomes more satisfyingly the patient's own rather than a matter of obedience to the therapist. [1965]

(In Erickson, 1980, Vol. IV, chap. 17, p. 190)

The writer recognizes that complete awareness of absolute truth is much less available than happy adjustments based upon those partial understandings acceptable to individuals and available and suitable to their own unique limitations. [circa 1950's]

(In Erickson, 1980, Vol. IV, chap. 40, p. 368)

The purpose of psychotherapy is to enable a patient to achieve a legitimate personal goal as advantageously as is possible. [circa 1930's]

(In Erickson, 1980, Vol. IV, chap. 54, p. 482)

It is imperative that recognition be given to the fact that comprehensive therapy is unacceptable to some patients. Their total pattern of adjustment is based upon the continuance of certain maladjustments which derive from actual frailties. Hence, any correction of those maladjustments would be undesirable if not actually impossible. Therefore, a proper therapeutic goal is one that aids the patient to function as adequately and constructively as possible under those internal and external handicaps that constitute a part of his life situation and needs.

(Erickson, 1954d, p. 109)

Indeed, it often seems absurd to attempt to reeducate patients when all that may be needed may be a redirection of their endeavors, rather than a change or a correction of their behavior. [1973]
(In Erickson, 1980, Vol. IV, chap. 38, p. 348)

Nor should therapists have so little regard for their patients that they fail to make allowance for human weaknesses and irrationality. [1965]
(In Erickson, 1980, Vol. IV, chap. 20, p. 212)

One does not try to force upon his patient a new pattern, but rather to reestablish the old unused and forgotten pattern of behavior the patient had previous to the development of his phobia.
(Erickson, 1941b, p. 17)

One takes the attitude that the patient is there to benefit *eventually* — perhaps in a day, a week, a month, six months, but within some reasonable period — *not* in the immediate moment. This tendency to correct the immediate behavior must be avoided because the patient really needs to show you that particular behavior.
(Erickson & Rossi, 1981, p. 18)

Focus on the Future, Not on the Past

Erickson was concerned only with the adequacy of a patient's present and future adjustments to reality. Insight into the mistakes of the past or into the past causes of present problems were of minor interest to him. He pointed out that the past is over and cannot be changed. His only concern with the past was that patients develop the ability to look at it carefully and objectively in order to overcome whatever misperceptions, or irrational beliefs, or limitations from the past were influencing their present behavior. He stated that insight into causal connections with prior events may be useful to the extent that it enables the therapist to guide the patient's attention toward relevant memories, but insight on the part of the patient was not the goal.

Insight into the past may be somewhat educational. But insight into the past isn't going to change the past. If you were jealous of your mother, it is always going to be a fact that you *were* jealous of her. If you were unduly fixated on your mother, it is always going to be the fact. You may have insight, but it doesn't change the fact. Your patient has to live in accord with things of today. So you orient your therapy to the patient living today and tomorrow, and hopefully next week and next year.
(Zeig, 1980, p. 269)

You have those learnings, in adult life, you can correct them. But there is no real need to correct them. They should be appreciated.
(Erickson, Rossi & Rossi, 1976, p. 214)

Well, the deed is done and cannot be undone, so let the dead past bury its dead. [1964]
(In Erickson, 1980, Vol. I, chap. 13, p. 325)

Emphasis should be placed more upon what the patient does in the present and will do in the future than upon a mere understanding of why some long-past event occurred.
(Erickson, 1954d, p. 127)

You present new ideas and new understandings and you relate them in some indisputable way to the remote future. **It is important to present therapeutic ideas and post hypnotic suggestions in a way that makes them con-**

tingent on something that will happen in the future.
(Erickson & Rossi, 1975, p. 148)

The rest of the hour was spent in an "explanation of the importance of reordering the behavior patterns for tomorrow, the next day, the next week, the next year, in brief, of the future, in order to meet the satisfactory goals in life that are desired." [1964]
(In Erickson, 1980, Vol. I, chap. 13, p. 315)

It's so ridiculous to pore over what you did when you were five years old because it belongs to the unchangeable past and any present understandings of that are different than that of the five year old. The adult level of understanding precludes any real understanding of the child's or the adolescent's world.
(Rossi, 1973, p. 15)

The problems were remote in origin, recent only in manifestation. To search for those remote origins would have been impossible until the traumatic course of stressful emotional events rendered the patients more accessible and probably more permanently damaged. Past experience with many similar patients suggests the importance of a ready approach to the immediate problem by dealing with it directly.
(Erickson & Rossi, 1979, p. 358)

Yes, take them from where they are now. That's where they are going to live today. Tomorrow, they live in tomorrow...next week, next month and next year. You might as well forget your past. Just as you forgot how you learned how to stand up, how you learned to walk, how you learned to talk. You have forgotten all that.
(Zeig, 1980, p. 221)

If your patient has something covered up, she's got it covered up for a very good reason, and you'd better respect that fact. You ask the patients to respect the fact that you personally do not think it needs to be covered up but that you are going to abide by their needs, *their actual needs.* Now you've told them you will abide by their needs, but they don't hear you qualify it to their "actual needs."

(Erickson & Rossi, 1979, p. 347)

It is essential that the therapist understand it [the patient's past] as fully as possible but without compelling the patient to achieve the same degree of special erudition. It is out of the therapist's understandings of the patient's past that better and more adequate ways are derived to help the patient to live his future.

(Erickson, 1954d, p. 128)

To assume that the original maladjustment must necessarily come forth again in some disturbing form is to assume that good learnings have neither intrinsic weight nor enduring qualities, and that the only persisting forces in life are the errors.

(Erickson, 1954d, p. 127)

From the point of view of analytic therapy, it is particularly interesting to emphasize that the obsessional phobia was relieved merely by the recovery of these specific conditioning events and without any investigation or discharge of underlying patterns of instinctual oedipus relationships, castration anxiety, or the like. [1939]

(In Erickson, 1980, Vol. III, chap. 23, p. 255)

Familiarity breeds contempt. When you go through a painful situation again and again in a dream, changing it a bit each time, it becomes less painful. [circa 1940's]

(In Erickson, 1980, Vol. IV, chap. 35, p. 334)

Objectivity Cures

Erickson noticed that people automatically respond more effectively when they are able to view the past, the present, and even the future in an objective, detached manner. As noted earlier, he attributed disordered or ineffectual behavior to a lack of exposure to accurate objective data about something, whether the environment, the past, or oneself. In a similar manner, he maintained that the provision of accurate, experientially based information or an objective appraisal would initiate growth-oriented responses from a majority of patients.

> **There is a natural tendency to overemphasize the importance of immediate understandings and subjective attitudes in preference to a thoughtful, objective consideration of eventual probabilities and possibilities. [circa 1940's]**
>
> *(In Erickson, 1980, Vol. IV, chap. 46, p. 424)*

> **This comprehensive, objective viewing of stressful matters is thus carried out against suggested backgrounds of various possible understandings. Ideally, objective thinking is possible in the ordinary waking state, but emotional stress is likely to constitute a serious interference, if not an actual barrier. [circa 1940's]**
>
> *(In Erickson 1980, Vol. IV, chap. 46, p. 424)*

> **The pressing emotional urgency of the actual current situation can be altered by the interjection or interpolation of a sense of perspective in time, thereby creating an opportunity conducive to more comprehensive and objective thinking. [circa 1940's]**
>
> *(In Erickson, 1980, vol. IV, chap. 46, p. 424)*

Thus he was enabled to see himself in an objective, detached fashion and, from unrecognized inner knowledge, to appreciate exactly what was occurring. [1937–38]

(In Erickson, 1980, Vol. IV, chap. 55, p. 493)

I gave Louise one nice look at her childish behavior. That was enough. I had her see her childish behavior in the behavior of other people who should know better. That was all the therapy that was needed.

(Zeig, 1980, p. 226)

Inducing and compelling an open-mindedness or mental receptiveness to new, inexplicable, curiosity-evoking ideas in settings causing the patient to look forward with hopeful anticipation and not to expend her energies in despondent despair over the past. [1963]

(In Erickson, 1980, Vol. IV, chap. 30, p. 311)

The overlay of neuroticism, however extensive, does not distort the central core of the personality, though it may disguise and cripple the manifestations of it. [1952]

(In Erickson, 1980, Vol. I, chap. 6, p. 146)

Objectivity Requires Reorganization

In order for patients to develop the more accurate and objective view of themselves and of reality that will enable them to cope more effectively, they obviously must change their present orientations toward that reality. This change in orientation was described by Erickson as a reordering, a resynthesis or a restructuring of the rigid and inhibiting conscious mental sets that patients have. *The initiation or facilitation of this restructuring process was his primary therapeutic goal.*

In some ways, Erickson was not concerned about where this restructuring began because he had discovered that once a patient experiences anything in a new way or from a new perspective, this new orientation will spread throughout the system. The destruction of any segment of a rigid and limiting mental set will initiate reverberating alterations and reassociations throughout the person's experiential life. Getting patients to experience something that would violate or disrupt their habitual conscious patterns of perception, thought, and response was what he wanted to accomplish. Once that had been accomplished, patients were allowed to grow and to develop in their own unique ways.

It is the experience of reassociating and reorganizing his own experiential life that eventuates in a cure, not the manifestation of responsive behavior which can, at best, satisfy only the observer. [1948]
(In Erickson, 1980, Vol. IV, chap. 4, p. 38)

Therapy results from an inner resynthesis of the patient's behavior achieved by the patient himself. [1948]
(In Erickson, 1980, Vol. IV, chap. 4, p. 38)

Not until he goes through the inner process of reassociating and reorganizing his experiential life can effective results occur. [1948]
(In Erickson, 1980, Vol. IV, chap. 4, p. 39)

The induction and maintenance of a trance serve only to provide a special psychological state in which the patient can reassociate and reorganize his inner psychological complexities and utilize his own capacities in a manner in accord with his own experiential life.... therapy

results from an *inner resynthesis* of the patient's behavior achieved by the patient himself. ...It is this experience of reassociating and reorganizing his own experiential life that eventuates in a cure. [1948]

(In Rossi, 1973, p. 19)

Hence, no more than was necessary was said to initiate those inner processes of her own behavior, responses and functionings which would be of service to her. [1964]

(In Erickson, 1980, Vol. I, chap. 13, p. 330)

It altered the place they could go for pleasure. It was a breakdown of a narrow, limited, restricted life existence. You can't be rigid in one area alone, it always spreads.

(Rossi, 1973, p. 15)

Providing the patient with alternatives sets the stage for inner search and creative problem-solving.

(Erickson, 1980, Vol. IV, p. 148)

To break her inhibitions, really break them! Notice how I engineered that: first the left shoe, then the right, the left stocking, then the right. I carefully built up a momentum of an affirmative character so she finally took off all her clothes and followed all my suggestions designed to shatter her lifelong inhibitions.

(Rossi, 1973, p. 13)

There results then a new psychological orientation of compelling force, effecting a new organization of thinking and planning. The writing of the letter constituted an initiation of action, and an action once initiated tends to continue.

(Erickson, 1954c, p. 283)

Thus he was placed in a situation permitting the development of a new frame of reference at variance with the repressed material of his life experience, but which would permit a reassociation, an elaboration, a reorganization, and an integration of his experiential life. [1948]
(In Erickson, 1980, Vol. IV, chap. 4, p. 43)

You always have patients experience as much of themselves and their limiting sets as possible within therapy. *The most important thing in therapy is to break up the patient's rigid and limiting mental sets.*
(Erickson & Rossi, 1979, p. 343)

I facilitate a certain flexibility in mental functioning when I remind her how easily her pleasure and fear can be "removed and reassumed."
(Erickson & Rossi, 1979, p. 347)

We are giving the patient new possibilities and we are taking away the undesirable qualities.
(Erickson & Rossi, 1979, p. 330)

And when I shattered that rigid idea it shattered the hell out of them. It even led them to try other positions. I hadn't told them there were other positions, they started investigating other positions on their own.
(Rossi, 1973, p. 15)

R: So you can actually enhance physical abilities by breaking through conscious bias about limitations.
E: Yes, unrecognized conscious bias.
(Erickson, Rossi & Rossi, 1976, p. 178)

Yes, it disrupted the rigidity that governed her entire life. Just as the first break in the shell pecked by a newly emerging chick immediately shatters the whole shell so

her whole life opened up. I just gave her simple statements. You do this, do that. No questions, just do it
silently.

(Rossi, 1973, p. 12)

He's placed a bad interpretation on a loss of erection.
Why should he keep that forever and ever?

(Erickson & Rossi, 1979, p. 266)

I am getting her away from her own habitual conscious
patterns.

(Erickson & Rossi, 1981, p. 80)

I'm asking her to adopt a frame of reference that is
totally new and different.

(Erickson & Rossi, 1979, p. 344)

R: That's the therapeutic response...
E: Yes, getting a new frame of reference.

(Erickson & Rossi, 1981, p. 255)

R: You are structuring a learning set for therapeutic
change.
E: Yes, new and different learnings for psychotherapeutic change. Without saying "Now I'm going to cram
down your throat some new understanding."

(Erickson, Rossi & Rossi, 1976, p. 33)

I want you to read the last chapter first and then you
sit down and try to think, wonder and speculate on what
was in the preceding chapter. Think in all directions, and
read that second to last chapter and see in how many
ways you were wrong; and you will be wrong in a lot of
ways. Then you read that second to the last chapter and
by the time you read a good book from the last chapter
to the first chapter, wondering and speculating, imagi-

ning, and figuring out, you'll learn to think freely in all directions.

(Zeig, 1980, p. 128)

The patient comes to you with a certain mental set and they expect you to get into that set. If you surprise them, they let loose of their mental set and you can frame another mental set for them.

(Erickson, Rossi & Rossi, 1976, p. 128)

When patients find something new, never again can they function in the old incomplete way. Their world is permanently changed.

(Erickson & Rossi, 1979, p. 392)

Therapy is often a matter of tipping the first domino. All that was needed was the correction of one behavior and if that one behavior was corrected....

(Rossi, 1973, p. 14)

Because once you break that restrictive, phobic pattern, the person will venture into other things.

(Zeig, 1980, p. 255)

When you get that wrongly directed energy turned in another direction, the patient heals.

(Zeig, 1980, p. 110)

When you get the patient to do the main work, all the rest of it falls in place.

(Zeig, 1980, p. 159)

You depend upon the patient's natural associative process to put things together.

(Erickson & Rossi, 1979, p. 386)

You start patients in a train of association, but they drift along on their own currents of thought and frequently leave the therapist stranded far behind.
(Erickson, Rossi & Rossi, 1976, p. 93)

This also gets the person into their own individuality. In psychotherapy we are looking for individualities. A patient, all too often, does not have much.
(Erickson & Rossi, 1979, p. 390)

R: **The cure is to let that individuality come out and flower in all its particular genius.**
E: **That's right. That's what you need to do, and that is why they are seeing you.**
(Erickson, Rossi & Rossi, 1976, p. 39)

You let the subject grow!
(Erickson, Rossi & Rossi, 1976, p. 265)

And remember always that you're unique. And all that you have to do is let people see that you are you.
(Erickson & Lustig, 1975, Vol. 2, p. 6)

Only Experiences Can Initiate Reorganization

As mentioned previously, people learn from experience. Only experientially acquired learning can be used to guide behavior and only internal or external events that are experienced directly can disrupt old patterns and initiate new ones. Reorganization or resynthesis, therefore, is the production of a new perspective as the result of new internal or external experiences. Generating such experiences and helping the patient become able to learn from them is the task of the therapist.

Erickson's verbal interactions with his patients were designed to initiate experiences which would facilitate the resynthesis process. He often worded reorganizational statements vaguely or even incorrectly so that patients would restate his basic points to themselves in a clearer, more correct, or more personally meaningful manner. By this device he was able to elicit an internal experience that would have more impact than something heard but not experienced in a personal way. Words, phrases, or statements that trigger internal responses or that touch upon and move attention toward one's own experiential background evidently have a more significant effect than those that are understood on an intellectual but not an experiential level.

Similarly, Erickson's frequent use of metaphors, analogies, and personal anecdotes apparently was *partially* motivated by the desire to force the patient to personalize the meaning of his words. The import of his statements could become an experiential event which then would be translated automatically by patients into terms related to their own thoughts and previous experiences. He believed that these strategies were more likely to convey a meaning that could be experienced and internalized by the listener than simple or direct statements of his basic points.

Patients can only respond out of their own life experiences.

(Erickson & Rossi, 1979, p. 258)

Therefore, his response could derive only from his own experiential associations and learned activities. [1938]
(In Erickson, 1980, Vol. II, chap. I, p. 9)

You give many examples so that patients are more likely to find one that's personally convincing and actually helps alter their behavior. The only things I say to you that cling are those that touch upon your experience in some way. You always study your patients for evidence that they are accepting what you say.

(Erickson & Rossi, 1979, p. 346)

Now when you want to prove something to a subject, and really prove it to them, try to let the proof come from within them. And let it come from within them in a most unexpected way. [1959]

(In Erickson, 1980, Vol. I, chap. 9, p. 239)

It is this internalization of the suggestion that makes it an effective agent in behavior change.

(Erickson & Rossi, 1975, p. 146)

You are avoiding saying to the subject but get the subject to say themselves.

(Erickson, Rossi & Rossi, 1976, p. 86)

There is a need to give the patient an earnest, compelling desire to protect and to respect that which is accepted. Therefore, let patients reword the presented ideas to please themselves. Then they become the patients' own ideas!

(Erickson & Rossi, 1979, p. 436)

To grasp such an analogy requires a creative effort on his part. Because it is his own creative effort, he is less likely to reject it than if it was simply thrust upon him as a direct statement.

(Erickson & Rossi, 1979, p. 259)

Behavior Generates Experiences

Although Erickson relied heavily upon the effects of verbal interaction in his therapy and teaching to initiate internal experiences, his ultimate goal was to get his patients and students to do something, *anything*, that would generate an experientially based challenge to their rigid, maladaptive, conscious patterns of response. Behavior provides experiences that cannot be easily overlooked.

It is at this point that his psychotherapeutic strategies often become difficult to understand or to imitate effectively. He used a variety of behavioral prescriptions for his clients, including climbing mountains, racing a bike, squirting water between the front teeth, eating a ham sandwich, and removing every stitch of clothing while standing in his office. Each of these behaviors had immediate and beneficial effects upon the patients involved and these benefits rapidly spread to all areas of their lives. Obviously, however, the behaviors themselves are not universally applicable as therapeutic interventions. They were selected and prescribed for individual patients because of the particular needs, personalities, and areas of conceptual rigidity of these patients. Climbing mountains or stripping off all of one's clothes are not magical techniques that would be effective with everyone. Erickson clearly stated that what he had patients do was only a relatively straightforward response to the needs and personalities of his patients.

Whether he used behavioral prescriptions or complex metaphors, he was simply attempting to get his patients to experience something that would force them to confront the reality of themselves and their situations either directly or symbolically. If the symbolism was appropriate and blatant enough or if the patient could be induced to undergo the experience directly, then the destruction of repressive barriers, rigidities, or biases would become a *fait accompli* and the process of reorganization would continue apace.

> It clearly illustrates the need and the value of actual behavior in enabling a patient to make therapeutic progress. [1935]
>
> *(In Erickson, 1980, Vol. IV, chap. 58, p. 521)*

> I believe that patients and students should do things. They learn better, remember better.
>
> *(Zeig, 1980, p. 72)*

> The important thing is not so much bookwork, following the rules you read in books. The important thing is to get the patient to do the things that are very, very good for him.
>
> *(Zeig, 1980, p. 195)*

> In psychotherapy for you, I want action and response not words, ideas, theories, concepts. I want responses, desirable, good, informative responses of action and change, not contemplation of change, but change and action of a constructive sort. [circa 1930's]
>
> *(In Erickson, 1980, Vol. IV, chap. 54, p. 484)*

> The thing to do is to get your patient, any way you wish, any way you can, to do something.
>
> *(Zeig, 1980, p. 143)*

> Then, as a result of some concrete or tangible performance, the patient develops a profound feeling that the repressive barriers have been broken, that the resistances have been overcome, that the communication is actually understandable and that its meaning can no longer be kept at a symbolic level.
>
> *(Erickson, 1954, p. 128)*

And I had them do something. And he got a new perspective upon life and she got a new perspective upon the boresomeness of something she didn't like.

(Zeig, 1980, p.148)

When you have a patient with some senseless phobia, sympathize with it, and somehow or other, get them to violate that phobia.

(Zeig, 1980, p. 253)

Leading the patient to, "See what I [the patient] can do," is much more effective than letting the patient see what things the therapist can do with or to the patient. [1963]

(In Erickson, 1980, Vol. IV, chap. 30, p. 291)

The rest of the hour was spent in an "explanation of the importance of reordering the behavior patterns for tomorrow, of the future, in order to meet the satisfactory goals in life that are desired." This was all in vague generalities, seemingly explanations, but actually cautious post-hypnotic suggestions, intended to be interpreted by him to fit his needs. [1964]

(In Erickson, 1980, Vol. I, chap. 13, p. 315)

After exploration of the underlying causes of her problem, the next step in therapy was to outline in great detail, with her help, the exact course of activity that she would have to follow to free herself from past rigidly established habitual patterns of behavior. [1952]

(In Erickson, 1980, Vol. I, chap. 6, p. 164)

Patients Can and Must Do the Therapy

Erickson's position with regard to the desired role of the patient was simple and direct. He maintained that the patient has the ability to do something that will be beneficial and that it is the patient's responsibility to do it. The therapist can create conditions conducive to change, can attempt to motivate the patient to change and can even provide a change-inducing experience, but change must occur within the patient. Change cannot be forced upon patients and patients cannot be expected to change in ways that are inappropriate for their needs or foreign to their experiential backgrounds. Unfortunately, this also implies that some patients cannot or will not experience change under any conditions the therapist can create. Therapists who keep the burden of responsibility for change on the shoulders of their patients will have less difficulty recognizing and accepting their impotence in such circumstances.

People come to you for help when they could furnish their own help.

(Zeig, 1980, p. 195)

Well, you've got a lot of things to help you. And keep them handy — handy in every possible way. And know that your own brain cell responses can meet your needs.

(Erickson & Lustig, 1975, Vol. 2, p. 5)

If you can utilize the great variety of brain cells that exist in the human being and depend upon them to function in their own way of thinking you can rely upon your patient to be able to furnish you with the ways and means and methods of dealing with intricate problems of everyday living.

(ASCH, 1980, Taped Lecture, 8/14/66)

Now the important thing for all of you is to recognize that when a patient comes in to you tremendously handicapped, how handicapped is he really? What brain cells does he have unused?

(ASCH, 1980, Taped Lecture, 7/16/65)

People do any number of things against themselves, and they do it in a very intelligent way to defeat themselves, to destroy themselves and that's what you need to know. Because if anybody can destroy the self intelligently then they can also use their brains to build things up intelligently.

(ASCH, 1980, Taped Lectures, 8/14/66)

Therapy for both was predicated upon the assumption that there is a strong normal tendency for the personality to adjust if given an opportunity. [1955]

(In Erickson, 1980, Vol. IV, chap. 56, p. 505)

The potentials within a person can restore well-being. [1970]

(In Erickson, 1980, Vol. IV, chap. 6, p. 58)

You reach an understanding that every happiness is earned and, if given to you, it's merited. Because there is no such thing as a free gift; you have to earn it or you have to merit it. And merit requires labor and effort on your part.

(Erickson & Lustig, 1975, Vol. 2, p. 4)

The burden of responsibility was hers, the means was hers. [1964]

(In Erickson, 1980, Vol. I, chap. 13, p. 325)

Whatever he does has to be on his own responsibility.

(Erickson & Rossi, 1981, p. 195)

The patient himself must put the recommended regime into action. [1957]

(In Erickson, 1980, Vol. IV, chap. 5, p. 49)

R: You are continually putting the responsibility for change back on the patient.

E: On to them always!

(Erickson, Rossi & Rossi, 1976, p. 37)

You never give the patient the impression that you must be constantly alert. You give them the impression that they are always sharing in the responsibility for the success of the work.

(Erickson, Rossi & Rossi, 1976, p. 264)

No matter what the author said, she was dependent upon her own resources only. **[1964]**

(In Erickson, 1980, Vol. I, chap. 13, p. 330)

"You're here to get whatever benefit you can get. And I think you're reasonably intelligent and if you exercise your intelligence you really ought to find some way of getting some kind of benefit. And I really don't care what kind of benefit you receive so long as you take the benefit that is available to *you*." Now I was able to give the burden upon her. *She* had to take the benefit that *she* could get, the benefit that she could derive from the situation. I challenged her intelligence.

(ASCH, 1980, Taped Lectures, 2/2/66)

She came to me with a problem, and I tell her she is going to have to do some thinking. And then I demonstrate to her exactly the kind of thinking.

(Erickson & Rossi, 1979, p. 210)

All therapy occurs within the patient, not between the therapist and patient.

(Erickson & Rossi, 1979, p. 160)

Bear in mind that it is the patient who is the important element.

(Haley, 1967, p. 535)

What your patient does and what he learns must be learned from within himself. There is not anything you can force into the patient.

(Haley, 1967, p. 535)

Reliance was placed upon the patient's own thinking and intelligence to make the proper psychological interpretation of her symptom when she became ready for that realization. [1944]

(In Erickson, 1980, Vol. IV, chap. 2, p. 25)

In a learning situation you have to do your own learning. I want you to learn a lot faster than I did, It took me about 30 years to learn, and there is no sense in that.

(Erickson, Rossi & Rossi, 1976, p. 264)

When I see patients, I really want them to do a great deal of thinking, because I don't know what's right for them. They have to reach that through an understanding of what they know, have experienced.

(Erickson & Lustig, 1975, Vol. 2, p. 5)

Yes, I think Joe's a very competent young man. I think he was competent in his psychotherapy. I think my competence lay in the fact that I knew enough to induce the trance and sit back and encourage Joe to follow out his own inclinations and understandings.

(ASCH, 1980, Taped Lecture, 8/14/66)

I gave that boy an understanding of his own capacity to be his own therapist. I told him "Never overextend yourself, just be cautious."

(ASCH, 1980, Taped Lecture, 8/14/66)

The experienced therapist makes clear to patients that responses must be in accord with their own potentialities, even though those potentialities may as yet be unrealized, misused, or misunderstood. [1973]
(In Erickson, 1980, Vol. IV, chap. 38, p. 348)

And some people love their illness and keep their illness, so you force them to do something to be frank.
(Zeig, 1980, p. 324)

There are some people you can't help. You can try.
(Zeig, 1980, p. 284)

Any young man who will impose upon his wife in the first seven years in that fashion is not going to change.
(Zeig, 1980, p. 201)

He is a born loser. Born to lose. Born to be a failure.
(Zeig, 1980, p. 210)

There is no hope for those people — they are professional patients. That is their sole goal in life.
(Zeig, 1980, p. 209)

There are other patients whose goal is no more than the continuous seeking of therapy but not the accepting of it. With this type of patient hypnotherapy fails as completely as do other forms of therapy. [1964]
(In Erickson, 1980, Vol. IV, chap. 19, p. 211)

Summary

Erickson emphasized the natural healing power of objectivity and avoided the seeking of insight. He accepted human imperfection but attacked and undermined conscious biases whenever they interfered with accurate objective awareness. His goal of psychotherapy was simple — a breakdown of biases to allow objectivity and freedom of action — but attainment of the goal often called for a complex restructuring of conscious understandings and responses. The initiation of these restructuring processes was accomplished by the creation of experiences, experiences that symbolically or indirectly moved patients toward more objective awareness of these abilities, thoughts, and situations. He generated internal experiences with his words and he generated external experiences with behavioral prescriptions. In all instances, however, he remained aware that the purpose of therapy is to allow patients to use their own potentials in whatever unique way is most productive and possible for them. Change, however, remains the patient's reponsibility. Some people cannot or will not be helped. Such is the reality of the therapy situation.

CHAPTER SIX

CREATING A PSYCHOTHERAPEUTIC CLIMATE

Although Erickson has been memorialized as a powerful and effective clinician who could cure even the most resistant or hopeless patients, he was exceedingly modest about the importance of the therapist within the therapy process. He challenged the "primacy of the therapist" attitude that pervades most other approaches and argued vehemently that it is the *patient's* needs, beliefs, abilities, and welfare which should define the character of therapy. He questioned the value and validity of pre-packaged, technique-oriented approaches to therapy that specify how a therapist should conduct a therapy session or what should be accomplished in therapy without reference to the individual patient. He rejected the use of a general theory to prescribe specific goals or techniques and he attacked the prejudices and professional inhibitions that often prevent therapists from recognizing or doing those things that are most responsive to a patient's needs.

In short, Erickson insisted that it must be the patient who
provides the goals, defines the process, and actually does the
therapy. Because he realized that it is up to the patient to undergo the desired changes, he recognized that the therapist can
do little more than provide a setting conducive to those
changes. The attitudes and behaviors necessary to create such
a setting were the subject of many of his comments and form
the bulk of the material contained in this chapter.

Therapists Provide Therapeutic Climates

According to Erickson, the therapist is a relatively unimpor-
tant component of the therapy process, merely the creator of a
catalytic situation. Thus, the first and most important thing
that a therapist can do is create a setting that will permit and
motivate patients to undergo the restructuring events necessary
to enable them to apply their experientially acquired learnings
effectively within a more objective view of themselves and of
the world. Therapists do not even have to know the nature of
the presenting problem or understand what needs to be done
to resolve it. All therapists really need to know is how to create a situation or relationship that will motivate patients to use
their own experiences and capacities to accomplish their own
therapy.

> I don't think the therapist is *the* important person; I
> think the patient is *the* important person in the situation.
>
> *(Erickson, 1977b, p. 22)*

> The therapist is really unimportant. It is his ability to
> get his patients to do their own thinking, their own un-
> derstanding.
>
> *(Zeig, 1980, p. 157)*

What the therapist knows, understands, or believes about a patient is frequently limited in character and often mistaken. What he is willing to let patients discover about themselves and to use effectively is of exceedingly great therapeutic importance. [1973]

(In Erickson, 1980, Vol. IV, chap. 38, p. 349)

It is the patient who does the therapy. The therapist only furnishes the climate, the weather. That's all. The patient has to do all the work.

(Zeig, 1980, p. 148)

I didn't know what her problem was. She didn't know what her problem was. I didn't know what kind of psychotherapy I was doing. All I was was a source of a weather or a garden in which her thoughts could grow and mature and do so without her knowledge.

(Zeig, 1980, p. 157)

I don't think the therapist does anything except provide the opportunity to think about your problem in a favorable climate.

(Zeig, 1980, p. 219)

I don't need to know what your problem is for you to correct it.

(Erickson & Rossi, 1979, p. 172)

The therapist merely stimulates the patient into activity, often not knowing what that activity may be, and then guides the patient and exercises clinical judgement in determining the amount of work to be done to achieve the desired results. [1948]

(In Erickson, 1980, Vol. IV, chap. 4, p. 39)

How to guide and to judge constitute the therapist's problem, while the patient's task is that of learning through his own efforts to understand his experiential life in a new way. [1948]

(In Erickson, 1980, Vol. IV, chap. 4, p. 39)

In psychotherapy you teach a patient to use a great many of the things that they learned, and learned a long time ago, and don't remember.

(Zeig, 1980, p. 38)

What they [therapists] say or do serves only as a means to stimulate and arouse in the subjects past learnings, understandings and experiential acquisitions, some consciously, some unconsciously acquired. [1964]

(In Erickson, 1980, Vol. I, chap. 13, p. 326)

What is needed is the development of a therapeutic situation permitting the patient to use his own thinking, his own understandings, his own emotions in the way that best fits him in his scheme of life. [1965]

(In Erickson, 1980, Vol. IV, chap. 20, p. 223)

I think that in hypnotherapy and in experimental work with subjects you have no right to express a preference; that it is a cooperative venture of some sort, and that the personality of the subject or the patient is the thing of primary importance. What the hypnotist or the therapist thinks, or does, or feels is not the important thing; but what he can do to enable the subject or the patient to accomplish certain things is important. It's the personality involved and the willingness of the therapist or the hypnotist to let the subject's personality play a significant role.

(Erickson, 1977a, p. 14)

> Thus, a favorable setting is evolved for the elicitation of needful and helpful behavioral potentialities not previously used, not fully used, or perhaps misused by the patient. [1966]
>
> *(In Erickson, 1980, Vol. IV, chap. 28, p. 263)*

Therapists Provide Motivation

Therapists do whatever is necessary to motivate patients. They serve as sources of comfort, hope, confidence, or inspiration and they serve as sources of frustration, discomfort, anger, and fear. They provide whatever it takes to initiate therapeutic movement. They do not instruct patients in the "proper" modes of thought or response; they merely create a therapeutic setting within which patients will be motivated, confident, and comfortable enough to do things that will help them discover, though their own experiences, whatever modes of thought or behavior are appropriate for their unique circumstances.

Erickson did not give pep talks to his patients to motivate them; he simply noticed the things that already motivated or interested them and used those. Once he had created a therapeutic atmosphere of trust, confidence, and an expectation of success, he could stimulate his patients into action using their natural sources of motivation as the trigger or impetus. More will be said about this crucial triggering component of the therapy process in the next chapter.

> The psychological aspect of medicine constitutes the art of medicine and transforms the physician from a skillful mechanic or technician into a needed human source of faith, hope, assistance, and, most importantly, of motivation toward physical and mental health and wellbeing. [1959]
>
> *(In Erickson, 1980, vol. IV, chap. 27, p. 255)*

He didn't need a direction about what to do. But he did need motivation. And that is one of the things in psychotherapy and the use of hypnosis — the motivation of a patient to do things. Not the things that you necessarily think they ought to do, but the things that they as personalities have the feeling that they really ought to do.

(Erickson & Rossi, 1981, p. 12)

When you talk toughly to the patient you give them an inspiration. They think they *can* do things. And you state it so simply and so earnestly you'd better believe what you are saying. How else are you going to get a patient who is despairing to do things? When you convey an understanding and an earnest and sincere belief.

(ASCH, 1980, Taped Lecture, 7/16/65)

My attitude towards patients is: You are going to accomplish your purpose, your goal. And I am very confident. I look confident. I act confident. I speak in a confident way, and my patient tends to believe me.

(Zeig, 1980, p. 61)

I was utterly confident. A good therapist should be utterly confident.

(Zeig, 1980, p. 61)

That is what my family says: "Why do your patients do the crazy things you tell them to do?" I say, "I tell it to them very seriously. They know I mean it. I am totally sincere. I am absolutely confident that they will do it. I never think, 'Will my patients do that ridiculous thing?' No, I know that they will."

(Zeig, 1980, p. 196)

Therapists Solicit Trust and Cooperation

In order to function as sources of inspiration, support, and motivation, therapists first must secure the trust and then the cooperation of patients. The atmosphere confronting a patient within the therapy setting must be conducive to the development of a sense of trust and cooperation. The essential ingredient of such an atmosphere is the therapist's genuine awareness of, respect for, and willingness to be responsive to the needs, fears, beliefs, and general personality of the patient. Patients do not enter therapy to be ridiculed, rejected, ignored, or dominated; they enter therapy to be protected, understood, and aided in their attempts to cope with the realities of their internal or external situations.

> **In dealing with patients, your entire purpose is to secure their cooperation and to make certain that they respond as well as they can.**
>
> *(Erickson & Rossi, 1981, p. 43)*

> **All techniques of procedure should be oriented about the subjects and their needs in order to secure their full cooperation. [1952]**
>
> *(In Erickson, 1980, Vol. I, chap. 6, p. 148)*

> **Merely to make a correct diagnosis of the illness and to know the correct method of treatment is not enough. Fully as important is that the patient be receptive of the therapy and cooperative in regard to it. Without the patient's full cooperativeness, therapeutic results are delayed, distorted, limited, or even prevented. [1965]**
>
> *(In Erickson, 1980, Vol. IV, chap. 20, p. 212)*

Actually, the real purpose was to develop in her a receptiveness, a responsiveness, a feeling of complete acceptance and a willingness to execute adequately any suggestion offered to her. [1965]

(In Erickson, 1980, Vol. IV, chap. 20, p. 220)

And, it is important to give them (*patients*) the opportunity of discovering that they can trust you.

(Erickson & Rossi, 1981, p. 5)

It is this that the patient comes in for, not to have the therapist take charge, but to give the therapist an opportunity of doing something, and doing something in accord with the needs of the patient, not in accord with the needs of the therapist.

(Erickson, 1977b, p. 22)

The primary problem is how to treat the patient so that his human needs may be met as much as possible. [1959]

(In Erickson, 1980, Vol. IV, chap. 27, p. 256)

In dealing with any type of patient clinically there is a most important consideration that should be kept constantly in mind. this is that the patient's needs as a human personality should be an ever-present question for the therapist to insure recognition at each manifestation. [1965]

(In Erickson, 1980, Vol. IV, chap. 20, p. 212)

That sense of goodness and adequacy is not to be based upon a sense of superiority of one's own attributes, but upon a respect for the self as an individual dealing rightfully with another individual, with each contributing a full share to a joint activity of significance to both. [1958]

(In Erickson, 1980, Vol. IV, chap. 15, p. 175)

Hence the therapist aids the patients to express quickly and freely their unpleasant feelings and attitudes, encouraging the patients by open receptiveness and attentiveness, and by the therapist's willingness to comment appropriately in a manner to elicit their feelings fully in the initial session. [1964]

(In Erickson, 1980, Vol. I, chap. 13, pp. 299–300)

Therapists Recognize and Accept Each Patient's Limitations

No therapist can create a therapeutic atmosphere if the realities of the patient's current condition are ignored, overlooked, or distorted. Therapists must learn to perceive and to respond to the reality confronting them, just as patients must.

Appearances and presentations aside, therefore, therapists must begin therapy with a full realization that the people they meet in therapy are not completely rational, sensible, or capable of responding in an adult manner to the obvious purposes of the situation. They may sound like reasonable and rational adults and they may present their problems in a manner that sounds mature, but the fact of the matter is that they are probably functioning in a very childish manner in many respects. This childish aspect of their functioning must be recognized and responded to if a therapeutic atmosphere is to be created. Unreasonable or childish beliefs and emotions should not be challenged as irrational, but must be respected and perhaps used. Patients should be treated with a certain amount of care and with a due consideration for and acceptance of all of the childish fears and foibles that they bring into therapy with them.

Too often the therapist regards patients as necessarily logical, understanding, in full possession of their faculties — in brief, as reasonable and informed human beings. [1965]

(In Erickson, 1980, Vol. IV, chap. 20, p. 212)

Nor should seemingly intelligent, rational, and cooperative behavior ever be allowed to mislead the therapist into an oversight of the fact that the patient is still human and hence easily the victim of fears and foibles, of all those unknown experiential learnings that have been relegated to his unconscious mind and that he may never become aware of or ever show just what the self may be like under the outward placid surface...Too often it is not the strengths of the person that are vital to the therapeutic situation. Rather, the dominant forces that control the entire situation may derive from weaknesses, illogical behavior, unreasonableness, and obviously false and misleading attitudes of various sorts. [1965]

(In Erickson, 1980, Vol. IV, chap. 20, p. 212)

But all of your patients have their own rigidities.

(Zeig, 1980, p. 121)

And our patients tend to restrict themselves and really cheat themselves out of a lot of things.

(Zeig, 1980, p. 255)

Patients often can't think for themselves. You start them thinking in some good reality way.

(Zeig, 1980, p. 288)

Patients can be silly, forgetful, absurd, unreasonable, illogical, incapable of acting with common sense, and very often governed and directed in their behavior by

emotions and by unknown, unrecognizable and perhaps undiscoverable unconscious needs and forces which are far from reasonable, logical, or sensible. [1965]
(In Erickson, 1980, Vol. IV, chap. 20, p. 212)

Adults are only little children grown a little older, and a lot taller. And they still behave like infants in the medical or dental or psychological office.
(ASCH, 1980, Taped Lecture, 7/16/65)

And another thing all patients should keep in mind, adults are only children grown tall.
(Erickson, Rossi & Rossi, 1976, p. 254)

So far as the patient is concerned you do not remind yourself of adult understandings. Nor do you look at behavior with adult understandings.
(Erickson, Rossi & Rossi, 1976, p. 215)

There was no other way for the patient to understand except in terms of intense childish beliefs and emotions with all their attitudes of acceptance.
(Erickson & Rossi, 1979, p. 435)

Such presentation [of ideas] needs to be in accord with the dignity of the patient's experiential background and life experience — there should be no talking down to, or over the head of, the patient. [1958]
(In Erickson, 1980, Vol. IV, chap. 15, p. 175)

Patients Are Ambivalent About Therapy

Patients enter the therapy setting with mixed emotions and conflicting desires. On the one hand they desire help and guidance, but on the other they are afraid to do what they know they must do. They may want nothing more than to have the therapist understand their situation perfectly, and yet they may do everything they can in order to hide their real problems or thoughts from the therapist.

Patients are people who have an injury; a painful, sore, uncomfortable, or embarrassing area of life. For one reason or another they have not been able to face these injuries and handicaps directly, which is why they have developed into problems. Accordingly, it is unreasonbable to expect patients to be willing or able to discuss their problems openly and objectively at first blush and it may be equally unreasonable and naive for therapists to believe what patients tell them initially. Therapists should not confuse the accepting attitude necessary for the creation of a therapeutic climate with absolute belief in what the patient says.

> **Every patient that walks into your office is a patient that has some kind of a problem. I think you'd better recognize that problem, that problems of all patients — whether they are pain, anxiety, phobias, insomnia — every one of those problems is a painful thing subjectively to that patient, only you spell the pain sometimes as p-a-i-n, sometimes you spell it p-h-o-b-i-a. Now, they're equally hurtful. And therefore, you ought to recognize the common identity of all of your patients. And your problem is, first of all, to take this human being and give him some form of comfort. And one of the first things you really ought to to is to let the patient discover where he really does have that pain...So that he can actually identify the pain and put it where it really belongs and not have it radiate to his total personality.**
>
> *(ASCH, 1980, Taped Lecture, 7/18/65)*

You should recognize that your patient is a totality whose toothache hurts clear down to the soles of his feet. And hurts clear back to the earliest learning that he acquired about how to grow up to be a big strong man. And that encompasses an awful lot of territory. And the same way with every other kind of distress.

(ASCH, 1980, Taped Lecture, 7/18/65)

Patients do come to you with tremendous anxiety. And it's all important that you recognize that anxiety, that you ought not to be led astray.

(ASCH, 1980, Taped Lecture, 2/2/66)

When a patient does a peculiar thing, when a patient gives a peculiar history, I think you ought to be very, very curious about it. Anxiety will show itself. You ought to be able to recognize it.

(ASCH, 1980, Taped Lecture, 2/2/66)

He [the patient] is both willing and unwilling to secure help from you.

(Erickson & Rossi, 1981, p. 4)

There always exists, whether recognized or not, a general questioning uncertainty about what will happen or what may or may not be said or done. [1952]

(In Erickson, 1980, Vol. I, chap. 6, p. 149)

They will hide that anxiety very carefully.

(ASCH, 1980, Taped Lecture, 2/2/66)

When you deal with patients they always want to hang onto something.

(Zeig, 1980, p. 93)

Any statesman can tell us that most of the world's troubles derive from a lack of communication. So it is with matters of human illness and health. [1970]

(In Erickson, 1980, Vol. IV, chap. 6, p. 75)

Mental disease is the breaking down of communication between people. [1970]

(In Erickson, 1980, Vol. IV, chap. 6, p. 75)

I think too often physicians overlook the meaningfulness of communication. They are listening to words, to stories, to general accounts and not listening to the actual communications that the patient is offering. And the actual communications concern the things that the patient is too afraid to face, too unwilling to face. That's why they are seeking professional help.

(ASCH, 1980, Taped Lecture, 2/2/66)

Why do patients have psychiatric problems? It's because they do not want to face them. Why do they have anxiety problems? Because they do not want to face the problems they have. And it's necessary for you to be willing to point out something. They want you to understand things that they do not know consciously that they are depending upon you to understand.

(ASCH, 1980, Taped Lecture, 2/2/66)

Now your patients come to you and tell you their problems. But do they tell you their problems or do they tell you what they *think* are problems? And are they problems only because they *think* that the things are problems?

(Zeig, 1980, p. 79)

How many patients come into your office convinced that this is the way it is and will be forever, when you in

your own knowledge know, "Yes, for a time you're going
to be depressed. But it's not forever."

(ASCH, 1980, Taped Lecture, 7/16/65)

Most neurotic ills come from people feeling inadequate, incompetent. And have they really measured their
competence?

(Zeig, 1980, p. 222)

Your patients in the psychiatric field are often exceedingly difficult. They are fearful to begin with, they are
distressed — they do not know how to handle themselves
or they would not be your patient.

(Erickson & Rossi, 1981, p. 8)

Patients Are Unreliable Sources

Even after the inhibiting anxieties of the first encounter
have diminished, what patients say during therapy should not
be accepted at face value. To do so is to ignore the obvious
fact that patients do not necessarily even know the most
important details about their situation and the added fact that
patients will try to protect themselves at all costs. Patients will
often lie, distort, conceal, rationalize, and resist all efforts to
help them. Such behavior may be childish and irrational, but it
is typical and, from the patient's perspective, necessary. Therapists who recognize the patient's need to engage in such tac-
tics will not be led astray by them and therapists who respect
or accept the validity of this need will not be infuriated or
frustrated by such avoidant actions. Recognition, acceptance,
and even utilization of whatever the patient presents will
accomplish far more than a narrow-minded or biased rejection
or challenge of it. Even the most sophisticated forms of resis-

tance and distortion can be used to create a therapeutic atmosphere of trust and cooperation if the therapist recognizes them and comprehends their necessity at the moment.

> **Even subjects who have unburdened themselves freely and without inhibition to the author as a psychiatrist have manifested this need to protect the self and to put their best foot forward no matter how freely the wrong foot has been exposed. [1952]**
>
> *(In Erickson, 1980, Vol. I, chap. 6, p. 149)*

> **Again the senior author reached the conclusion that the psychiatric portrayal she offered of herself was no more than a symptomatic screen to conceal her actual problem.**
>
> *(Erickson & Rossi, 1979, p. 444)*

> **And yet I do know that patients will conceal things.**
>
> *(ASCH, 1980, Taped Lecture, 2/2/66)*

> **Now, when a patient comes in you ought to be aware of the fact that the patient cannot face certain things at all and they are going to distract you. This matter of anxiety, they may distract you because they are resistant.**
>
> *(ASCH, 1980, Taped Lecture, 2/2/66)*

> **Patients come to you for help. They may resist help, but they hope desperately you'll win.**
>
> *(Zeig, 1980, p. 333)*

> **Now then, patients can resist and they will resist.**
>
> *(Zeig, 1980, p. 93)*

> **This adverse attitude [resistance] is part and parcel of their reason for seeking therapy; it is the manifestation of their neurotic attitude against the acceptance of therapy and their uncertainty about their loss of their defenses**

and hence it is a part of their symptomatology. Therefore this attitude should be respected rather than regarded as an active and deliberate or even unconscious intention to oppose the therapist. Such resistance should be openly accepted, in fact graciously accepted since it is a vitally important communication of a part of their problems and often can be used as an opening into their defenses. This is something that the patients do not realize; rather they may be distressed emotionally since they often interpret their behavior as uncontrollable, unpleasant, uncooperative rather than as an informative exposition of certain of their important needs. [1964]

(In Erickson, 1980, Vol. I, chap. 13, p. 299)

Often patients come to you not knowing why they are unhappy or distressed or disturbed in any way. All they know is that they are unhappy, and they give you a wealth of rationalizations to explain it.

(Erickson & Rossi, 1981, p. 7)

Consciously they will tell you any story that seems to be reasonable, that seems to be well founded. And they'll tell it to you with great intensity. They will make you believe it. But they are using that particular thing.

(ASCH, 1980, Taped Lecture, 2/2/66)

A person seeking therapy comes in and tells you one story that is believed fully at the conscious level and in nonverbal language can give you a story that is entirely different.

(Erickson, Rossi & Rossi, 1976, p. 68)

The patient is going to come in and withhold some vital information, tremendously vital information. And you see them laboriously sit down and assume a certain position that you have come to recognize as meaning

"I'm going to tell you everything except..." You'd better know that they're telling you everything except... and you'd better respect that and you'd better tell them right away "Now, while I expect you to tell me your entire history, certainly I don't want you to do it *today*. I want you to be willing to withhold a certain thing *until* you are really ready to tell me *more*.

(ASCH, 1980, Taped Lecture, 7/16/65)

Now I cite these two cases as actual instances of the need to listen to patients, always, and to form your own conclusions, and to form your conclusions from what *you* notice, from what *you* see, from what you understand and *never* to take your patient's word for anything.

(ASCH, 1980, Taped Lecture, 2/2/66)

Therapists Must Decipher What Patients Say

No matter what patients say, even if they are being as open and honest as possible and even if what they say makes perfect sense to the therapist, the wise therapist realizes the necessary gap between the real meaning of the patient's verbalizations and the perceived meaning. In order to avoid misunderstandings and misinterpretations, therapists should reserve judgement or belief until they are certain that they understand the personal meanings of the patient's vocabulary. As indicated previously, every person has a different perspective or orientation to the world and each underlying perspective gives words a slightly different meaning. Understanding can occur only after the therapist has managed to adopt the perspective of the patient and has listened to the patient's words and observed the patient's behavior from that perspective.

This is not an easy task. Adopting someone else's orientation to the world and seeing events from that perspective requires considerable effort, close attention, and continual practice. The conceptual flexibility required does not come automatically but must be developed by the therapist through continual practice.

To complicate matters further, the actual meaning of a communication or a behavior may reside within the patient's unconscious. Patients may say one thing at a conscious level and be oblivious to the unconscious communications inherent in their phrasings or intonations. The therapist's task, therefore, is not only to determine and adopt the patient's conscious perspectives and to decipher the meanings of communications from that orientation, but also to assume the orientation or framework of the patient's unconscious and to respond to the meanings of communications from that level of functioning as well.

The patterns or orientations of the unconscious are almost universal, which means that a therapist's unconscious probably can comprehend and respond to the meaning of the communications from the patient's unconscious reasonably well with little or no training. The difficulty, of course, lies in nurturing the therapist's ability to do so at a conscious level. Erickson's ability to do this may be attributable, in part, to his physiological anomalies which prevented him from being distracted by irrelevancies and, in part, to the years he spent carefully observing patients in order to learn the meanings of these unconscious verbal and nonverbal signals. Perhaps the only potential shortcut to the process of gaining increased access to the perceptions and understandings of the patient's unconscious is hypnosis. As will be discussed later, hypnosis can facilitate the therapist's understandings of and responses to the messages sent by the patient's unconscious.

Even if therapists do not fully comprehend the exact meaning of the patient's words or behaviors, the simple expedient of adopting the dominant or significant verbal and non-verbal mannerisms of the patient can provide the patient with a sense of comfort and understanding. The patient's concepts and vocabulary, not those of the therapist, should dominate the situation. As the therapist utilizes the patient's style of communication to convey meaning, the patient begins to feel understood, secure, and relieved of the burden of deciphering what the therapist says. A therapeutic atmosphere results and cooperation increases.

> **I never believe anything that I hear from that chair over there until I've confirmed and reaffirmed it. 'Cause it is interesting to listen to but you should not believe it until you really know. And that sort of an attitude toward your patients is utterly important.**
>
> *(ASCH, 1980, Taped Lecture, 2/2/66)*

> **Now I have the right to be as stupid as possible. It isn't requisite for me to understand all. There can be progressive understanding on your part.**
>
> *(Erickson, Rossi & Rossi, 1976, p. 132)*

> **I don't have to believe anything that anybody tells me. I don't believe it until I understand her words.**
>
> *(Zeig, 1980, p. 158)*

> **Whenever you see patients, you really ought to consider, "What type of orientation do they have?"**
>
> *(Zeig, 1980, p. 232)*

> **Every patient poses problems that need understanding from more than one point of view. [1957]**
>
> *(In Erickson 1980, Vol. IV, chap. 5, p. 51)*

You have to look at your patient as if you were sitting on a seat higher than his. You also have to look at him from a much lower seat. You need to look at him from the other side of the room. Because you always get a totally different picture from different points of view. Only by such a total look at the patient can you gain some objectivity.

(Erickson, Rossi & Rossi, 1976, p. 212)

Your approach to him must be in terms of him as a person with a particular frame of reference for that day and the immediate situation.

(Haley, 1967, p. 535)

And when you listen to the patient, listen to what you hear, then get over in that chair and listen again, because there is another side to the story.

(Zeig, 1980, p. 169)

When you listen to patients, listen carefully and try to think what is the other side of the story. Because if you just hear the patient's story, you really don't know all the story.

(Zeig, 1980, p. 169)

And so, your patients tell you many things and your tendency is to put your meaning upon the patient's words.

(Zeig, 1980, p. 174)

So, I warn all of you, don't ever, when you are listening to a patient, think you understand the patient, because you're listening with your ears and thinking with your own vocabulary. The patient's vocabulary is something entirely different.

(Zeig, 1980, p. 58)

And in psychotherapy you listen to your patient knowing that you don't understand the personal meaning of his vocabulary.

(Zeig, 1980, p. 158)

Now in psychotherapy — if you want to do psychotherapy — you have to learn, first of all, that each of us has a different meaning to the words used in common.

(Zeig, 1980, p. 173)

When you are doing psychotherapy, you listen to what the patients say, you use their words, and you can understand those words. You can place your own meaning on those words, but the real question is what is the meaning that a patient places on those words. You cannot know because you do not know the patient's frame of reference.

(Erickson & Rossi, 1981, p. 255)

So you listen to your patient knowing he has personal meaning for his words and you don't know his personal meaning. And he doesn't know your personal meanings for words. You try to understand the patient's words as *he* understands them.

(Zeig, 1980, p. 158)

I emphasized the importance of understanding the patient's words and really understanding them. You don't interpret your patient's words in *your* language.

(Zieg, 1980, p. 78)

I usually do not take a complete history. I want to listen to that first presentation that the patient offers.

(ASCH, 1980, Taped Lecture, 2/2/66)

You let the patients use their own words to describe the process.

(Erickson & Rossi, 1979, p. 381)

You search out for those things that are peculiar to the person.

(Erickson & Rossi, 1981, p. 100

Never forget folk language. You should always recognize how the folk language is related to symptom formation.

(Erickson & Rossi, 1979, p. 277)

The method by which a story is told may be even more important than its content. [1944]

(In Erickson, 1980, Vol. III, chap. 29, p. 355)

I hope I've taught you something about psychotherapy. The importance of seeing and hearing and understanding, and getting your patient to do something.

(Zeig, 1980, p. 158)

How many times does a patient need to state his complaint? Only that number of times requisite for the therapist to understand. [1966]

(In Erickson, 1980, Vol. IV, chap. 28, p. 277)

Yet experience has taught me the importance of my assumption of the role of a purely passive inquirer, one who asks questions solely to receive an answer regardless of its content. An intonation of interest in the meaning of the answer is likely to induce subjects to respond as if they had been given instructions concerning what answer to give. [1965]

(In Erickson, 1980, Vol. I, chap. 3, p. 94)

Therapists Must Acknowledge the Patient's Reality

There is a natural tendency, perhaps, to downplay the seriousness of a patient's condition or to employ euphemisms when referring to the more unpleasant and painful aspects of the situation. However, an important part of all patients' desires to be understood and accepted is the desire to find someone who will be honest with them, someone who will acknowledge with brutal frankness the validity of their accurate perceptions. This does not mean that their irrational fears and irrational beliefs must be given credence, but it does mean that the therapists should not argue with them and obviously should agree fully when there is some truth to what they say. The therapy situation must be an island of truth, a setting wherein two people can be honest with each other. Patients trust therapists who tell them the truth, though it must be remembered that it is largely the patient who determines what is true and what is not. Almost everything Erickson ever said to his patients was either an axiomatic, necessary truism, an objectively verifiable fact, or something that the patient already believed to be true. The development of trust depends upon honesty and acceptance. Once patients have learned that the therapist can be trusted, then the therapist can begin to direct them toward topics and experiences that they otherwise would have avoided.

She wanted understanding and recognition; not a falsification, however well-intended, of a reality comprehensible to her. [1958]

(In Erickson, 1980, Vol. IV, chap. 15, p. 176)

At no time was he given a false statement, nor was he forcibly reassured in a manner contradictory to his understandings. [1958]

(In Erickson, 1980, Vol. IV, chap. 15, p. 179)

He was told seriously and impressively, "You are entirely right, absolutely right..." [1965]

(In Erickson, 1980, Vol. IV, Chapter 20, p. 217)

Such a brutal beginning, with such negative statements only partially balanced by a final qualified favorable statement, could have no other effect than to convince her of my utter sincerity of purpose.

(Erickson & Rossi, 1979, p. 432)

That is a fact and you pause to let them reflect on the factual nature of that statement. They have a chance to recognize that you are really speaking the truth.

(Erickson, Rossi & Rossi, 1976, p. 39)

Calling a spade a spade, especially in the patient's own language, however unrecognized at the time, often expedites therapy by convincing the patient that the therapist is unafraid of his task and recognizes it clearly.

(Erickson & Rossi, 1979, p. 433)

If you're afraid ever to say a word or to name a condition to a patient, you're going to alert the patient to the fact that you are afraid.

(ASCH, 1980, Taped Lecture, 2/2/66)

But this matter of using metaphors, analogies, allegorical statements and so on to direct your patient's attention from one mood to another — and you never avoid what the patient says.

(ASCH, 1980, Taped Lecture, 7/16/65)

There is no more important problem than so speaking to the patient that he can agree with you and respect your intelligent grasp of the situation as judged by him in terms of his own understandings. [1958]
(In Erickson, 1980, Vol. IV, chap. 15, p. 177)

Every care was taken to ensure the desired understanding of it by the patient.
(Erickson, 1954d, p. 110)

You see, all I want to do is *to find out if we can understand each other.* [1964]
(In Erickson, 1980, Vol. I, chap. 13, p. 319)

Therefore he could listen respectfully to me, because I had demonstrated that I understood the situation fully. [1958]
(In Erickson, 1980, Vol. IV, chap. 15, p. 177)

A community of understandings was first established with him, and then, one by one, items of vital interest to him in his situation were thoughtfully considered and decided, either to his satisfaction or sufficiently agreeably to merit his acceptance. His role in the entire situation was that of an interested participant, and adequate response was made to each idea suggested. [1958]
(In Erickson, 1980, Vol. IV, chap. 15, p. 179)

I am taking over control of the total situation. I haven't offered anything with which he can take issue.
(Erickson & Rossi, 1981, p. 183)

Therapists Protect Patients

By accepting, understanding, and utilizing the productions of the patient, the therapist expresses a genuine concern and respect for the personality and needs of another individual.

Therapists must protect patients in every way possible rather than challenging or threatening them. Patients will relax and place their trust in a therapist who respects them and protects them by not expecting more from them than they can produce. Therapy will occur only if the therapist allows it and allows it to occur in a protective atmosphere as slowly or quickly as is necessary for the patient.

> All this is an introduction to one important thing, and I think it is paramount in any approach to hypnotic therapy. That is that one must always protect the subject or the patient. The patient does not come to you just because you are a therapist. The patient comes to be protected or helped in some regard. But the personality is very vital to the person, and he doesn't want you to do too much, he does not want you to do it too suddenly. You've got to do it slowly, you've got to do it gradually, and you've got to do it in the order in which he can assimilate it.
>
> *(Erickson, 1977b, p. 20)*

> There is a tremendous need for protecting patients in ordinary psychotherapy. How often is the resistance the result of the therapist's intruding upon intimate memories, intimate ideas? This accounts for a great deal of resistance, and in hypnotherapy one can reach that sort of situation by stating to the patients very definitely your intention to protect them.
>
> *(Erickson, 1977b, p. 34)*

> By emphasizing that she should reveal only what she can share with strangers, I'm keeping her on the surface. I'm protecting her.
>
> *(Erickson & Rossi, 1979, p. 373)*

> **There is a tremendous need for protecting patients in ordinary psychotherapy...And you should not overlook the possibility that you can unwittingly intrude upon the legitimate privacy of a patient.**
>
> *(Erickson, 1977b, p. 34)*

> **In a situation where one feels seriously damaged, there is an overwhelming need for a compensatory feeling of satisfying goodness. [1958]**
>
> *(In Erickson, 1980, Vol. IV, chap. 15, p. 178)*

Therapists Must Give Freedom to Patients

In order to avoid imposing unwarranted demands upon the patient and to provide the patient with a feeling of comfort and trust, the therapist must give the patient complete freedom, or at least the illusion of complete freedom. Even when purposefully guiding the patient's attention in a particular direction, the therapist must provide a variety of alternative paths toward that end. Patients should not feel the need to do exactly what the therapist wants, but should feel free to respond in whatever manner is most comfortable or natural and should be reassured that their responses are good. The feeling of freedom is one of the most pleasant and comforting of feelings, and the therapist's permissive attitude should convey this feeling continuously.

In some respects, this is simply a restatement of previous propositions regarding the creation of a therapeutic setting. The essential message provided by a general recognition, acceptance, and utilization of whatever the patient presents is one of freedom. Patients should be given permission to be whatever they are and thus the therapist should promote their freedom and provide protection for them. Any therapist who enters therapy with this attitude and who responds to patients in a manner that conveys it, will generate trust and cooperation.

It is desirable to do it indirectly, so that the patient does not feel under attack. It is a way of obviating defenses.

(Erickson & Rossi, 1979, p. 386)

You ought to have your techniques so worded that there are escape routes for all resistances — intellectual, emotional, situational.

(Erickson & Rossi, 1981, p. 221)

Let there be no hint of arbitrary demands, since the patient is resistant and this suggestion is one of freedom of response, even though of an illusory freedom. [1964]

(In Erickson, 1980, Vol. I, chap. 13, p. 306)

The common mistake in psychotherapy is to give a patient directions without recognizing there have to be doubts.

(Erickson, Rossi & Rossi, 1976, p. 216)

And so when a patient comes to me, I have all the doubts, I doubt in the right directions. The patient doubts in the wrong direction.

(Zeig, 1980, p. 46)

And nobody can control you, you can defy me any time you want to, or anybody else. You are a free citizen, and be free with yourself.

(Erickson & Rossi, 1979, p. 232)

In therapy this is often the way you get patients to become more aware of their capabilities. You are essen-

tially giving them the freedom to use themselves. Patients come to you because they don't feel free to use themselves.
(Erickson, Rossi & Rossi, 1976, p. 292)

Yes, you always depontentiate her doubts by giving her many possible modes of response.
(Erickson & Rossi, 1979, p. 413)

Your attitude should be completely permissive [1976–78]
(In Erickson, 1980, Vol. I, chap. 23, p. 486)

You only interfere when they try to destroy themselves.
(Erickson & Rossi, 1981, p. 12)

You see, psychologically one needs to give the patient the opportunity both to accept and reject anything you offer. [1976–78]
(In Erickson, 1980, Vol. I, chap. 23, p. 483)

She has a tremendous amount of freedom to explore all these possibilities in her past — and all this by implication.
(Erickson & Rossi, 1979, p. 413)

I give him a feeling of choice even though I'm determining it.
(Erickson & Rossi, 1981, p. 224)

I'm giving her freedom...
(Erickson & Rossi, 1979, p. 199)

I like to *approach* my psychiatric patients — whether they are neurotic, emotionally disturbed, prepsychotic or even psychotic — in a fashion that lets them *feel free to respond to whatever degree they wish.*
(Erickson & Rossi, 1981, p. 4)

That's right. You create a situation in which they can move and respond freely, comfortably, safely, securely.

(ASCH, 1980, Taped Lecture, 7/16/65)

You don't want your patients to feel as if they are under a great burden, so I carefully give her a chance to give this answer.

(Erickson & Rossi, 1979, p. 383)

The Patient's Welfare is the Only Concern

The conduct and content of therapy should reflect only the needs and personality of the patient because the welfare of that patient, i.e. his or her freedom, benefit, and protection, should be the only considerations in the therapist's office. Other considerations that too often enter into the conduct of therapy and displace an awareness of or a responsiveness to the needs of the patient include: the therapist's concern with his or her own prestige or professional image, social conventions or etiquette, and even common courtesy or social niceties. None of these issues should inhibit therapists from doing whatever is necessary to promote the welfare of their patients. Therapists must be willing to look foolish at times, to behave "inappropriately" at others and, in general, to ignore or overlook a "what-will-people-think" attitude.

Erickson had only one concern, the welfare of his patients, and he said or did whatever he judged to be necessary to maximize that welfare without regard for other concerns. By refusing to allow irrelevancies to inhibit his therapeutic style, he was able to create a totally new concept of the therapy process. He put the patient's unique concerns and needs in the central spotlight and he kept them there from the beginning to the end of therapy. His willingness and ability to do this were based upon his recognition of the necessity for doing it, and his recognition of the necessity for doing it gave form and substance to his entire therapeutic strategy. He used what the patient brought into the office and he did not demand or expect more than the patient had to offer or could accomplish.

On the other hand, his concern with his patients' welfare did not prevent him from doing things that were embarrassing or upsetting to them if that was what was necessary to motivate them to use their potentials and understand their experiences. He was concerned with his patients' welfare, but not with being liked or respected by them. He comforted his patients, but not when their welfare required otherwise. The patient's protection and welfare supersede all other general considerations, which makes specific rules of therapy difficult. In a sense, almost anything goes as long as patients are protected and their welfare is promoted. This maxim could be used to justify some pretty strange or totally inappropriate activities, but it does not apply unless patients actually derive benefit from those activities and unless the therapist actually has the patients' protection and welfare at heart. It may seem cruel to intentionally frustrate a brain-damaged patient, but Erickson did so in order to motivate compensatory learning. It may seem inappropriate to have an embarrassed young woman strip, point to and name every part of her body, but Erickson did so to break through her devastating inhibitions and rigidities. In every situation, however, he ensured that the rights and personalities of his patients were completely protected in some obvious manner. He did what he had to do *for their benefit*. He let them react to him in whatever way they needed to *for their benefit*. He even let them pay what they needed to *for their benefit*. The patient's welfare, not the therapist's, was his primary concern.

I think you ought always to recognize your patient as a totality, as a person, as a person with a personality, as a person that thinks and feels and believes and wants, and who understands certain things to a certain degree, and that your task is to communicate with him in a way that gives him the ideas and the understandings that he wants and needs, and to ask him to do some thinking on his own so that he can correct any misunderstandings. That he should participate with you in achieving a goal in common. His welfare, not your welfare, not the establishment of your professional eminence or anything of that sort, but his *welfare*. And your orientation to the patient as a person whose welfare you are interested in is the important thing.

(ASCH, 1980, Taped Lecture, 7/16/65)

Her welfare was the governing purpose of the therapy devised—not sympathy, consideration, or even common courtesy. [1964]

(In Erickson, 1980, Vol. IV, chap. 30, p. 310)

They were all deliberately and intentionally controlled and directed *toward the evoking of whatever capacities for all kinds of responses which she might have or could develop*, without regard for courtesies or social niceties, *but only for whatever responsive behavior might be conducive to restoration of previous patterns of normal behavior.* [1964]

(In Erickson, 1980, Vol. IV, chap. 30, p. 310)

The kind of therapy warranted should be that which is considered clinically to meet the patient's needs and to offer the best possible therapeutic results without regard for social niceties or questions of etiquette. There should be only one ruling principle — the patient's welfare.

(Erickson, 1980, Vol. 4, p. xxi)

Yet medical problems, whatever they are, should be faced, and patients' needs should be met without regard for irrelevant social teachings.

(Erickson, 1980, Vol. IV, p. xxii)

One's professional dignity is not involved but one's professional competence is. [1965]

(In Erickson, 1980, Vol. IV, chap. 30, p. 213)

You see, I think the important thing in working with a patient is do the thing that is going to help the patient. As for my dignity ... the hell with my dignity. (Laughs) I will get along all right in this world. I don't have to be dignified, professional. I do the thing that stirs the patient into doing the right thing.

(Zeig, 1980, p. 143)

Therapy is going to be socially oriented, that the emotional and social needs will be the prime consideration, and that while I may be seemingly offensive, there is a worthy principle involved.

(Erickson & Rossi, 1979, p. 276)

I don't like these physicians who wear a high silk hat and a starched front to their shirt and a fresh suit to the office and very, very professional manner and all that sort of thing. The office is where two human beings meet to solve a problem and I think that you can be a human being and abide by professional ethics and professional courtesy in every way and still be human, so that they know you are and so that they can confide in you. I think that's one of the most important things.

(ASCH, 1980, Taped Lecture, 7/16/65)

My approach is very casual even with this difficult material, and that makes it easier for her. It's hard to say "no" to a casual easygoing approach.

(Erickson & Rossi, 1979, p. 322)

You keep things informal so you give the patient the privilege of concealing just how important some of these things are.

(Erickson & Rossi, 1979, p. 371)

Now, that letting loose — why did she? I set an example of relaxation, of comfort, of actually enjoying her presence no matter how rigid she was, until she had a feeling of comfort out of the situation.

(ASCH, 1980, Taped Lecture, 7/16/65)

I always sprawl out in my chair because I like to be comfortable. In fact I have to be comfortable. And so I sprawl out.

(ASCH, 1980, Taped Lecture, 7/16/65)

In teaching, in therapy, you are very careful to use humor, because patients bring in enough grief, and they don't need all that grief and sorrow. You better get them in a better frame of mind right away.

(Zeig, 1980, p. 71)

In presenting therapeutic understandings a little roughage, as in the diet, is essential. Therapists who insist that everything they present is good and acceptable — and must be accepted because it is always tendered in courteous language and manner — are in error.

(Erickson & Rossi, 1979, p. 436)

However farcical the above procedure may seem in itself, it possessed the remarkable and rare virtue of being satisfying to the patient as a person and meeting his symptomatic needs adequately.

(Erickson, 1954d, p. 111)

This thinking led to extensive experimentation by deliberately making out-of-character, irrelevant, nonsequitur remarks in groups and to single persons. [1964]
(In Erickson, 1980, Vol. I, chap. 10, p. 261)

When you seem to be doing damn fool things, it takes your patient's mind off his pain.
(Zeig, 1980, p. 292)

The primary task in the therapy of various psychopathological conditions may be dependent upon an approach seemingly unrelated to the actual problem. [1943]
(In Erickson, 1980, Vol. II, chap. 14, p. 156)

The goal sought is often infinitely more apparent than the apparent logic of the procedure. [1952]
(In Erickson, 1980, Vol. I, chap. 6, p. 144)

She looked at me as though she thought I ought to have my head examined.
(Erickson, 1977b, p. 31)

I asked him to repeat my name until he wondered who was the patient.
(Erickson, 1977b, p. 22)

There's iron under my velvet gloves.
(Rossi, 1973, p. 14)

Summary

Erickson created an environment wherein patients were encouraged to use their experiences to grow and to develop in whatever manner was suitable for them. As a consequence, they were able to accept the responsibility for change and to feel comfortable enough to risk changing. The creation of such a setting is what being a therapist is all about from Erickson's perspective. Therapists must turn their attention away from themselves, away from their own needs, their own expectations, their professional images, and their evaluation by others. They must direct their attention solely and totally toward the patient because it is the patient whose cooperation is needed to provide the necessary experiences, understandings, and changes. Because each patient is unique, the form of intervention or the type of change required is unique as well. Only patients themselves can provide the specific information or alterations necessary and they will not be able to do so effectively if the therapist fails to create a therapeutic setting — a setting wherein the patient's needs, thoughts, and deeds are primary and where the patient feels understood, accepted, protected, and willing to cooperate.

CHAPTER SEVEN

INITIATING THERAPEUTIC CHANGE

Although there are times when the mere provision of a therapeutic climate will initiate therapeutic change, this is the exception rather than the rule. More typically, the creation of a therapeutic change can then be initiated by appropriate interventions. A therapeutic climate allows the patient to provide the therapist with useful information and makes the patient more willing and able to act upon or respond to the interventions eventually offered by the therapist. The actual change process itself, however, is usually initiated by an experience that occurs within the context of the therapeutic climate and not by the therapeutic climate *per se*.

Erickson argued that therapy itself is accomplished when patients experience something (preferably as a result of actually doing something themselves to cause that experience) which, in some unknown manner, triggers a reorganization or resynthesis and new applications of previous understandings and responses. Such a change-initiating experience may involve the behavioral or perceptual violation of a previously held falsehood, misperception, or rigid restriction or it may simply involve the presentation of the truth of the matter to the patient in a direct, a metaphoric, or a symbolic manner. In some instances, therapeutic change results when patients are provided with a demonstration of skills or abilities they did not believe they had.

Although this may sound like a fairly simple assignment for the therapist, it must be remembered that patients are people who cannot or will not recognize the truth or utilize their experiences and capacities fully. They have and will continue to resist change. They must be propelled into accepting change somehow, not merely asked to do so.

Erickson was a master at generating such propulsions. He consistently discovered aspects of the patient's unique patterns of interest, thought, emotion, or behavior that could be redirected to create an experience that would undermine the undesirable, inappropriate, or limiting conditions brought into the office by that patient and he did so in ways that the patient could not and would not escape. He challenged one patient to a bicycle race in order to create an experience that would prove her capabilities to her. He had a couple compare their reactions to climbing a mountain in order to force them to recognize their basic personality differences. He taught a boy to read by looking at maps of potential vacation spots with him. He motivated neurologically impaired individuals to relearn how to do things by being impolite, by frustrating them, or even by infuriating them. He grabbed hold of whatever unique interests or primary qualities a person brought into the office and he utilized them in ways that would enable his patients to accomplish their purposes.

Erickson's focus upon the unique qualities of each patient

and his remarkable ability to utilize whatever unique attributes he observed in order to stimulate therapeutic change are the central considerations of this chapter. The purpose of the following material is to convey the basic attitude underlying his utilization approach. However, a genuine appreciation for the mechanics of Erickson's utilization techniques will probably not be possible until the reader has also reviewed several of his case examples in detail. Thus, the summary of a number of his therapy cases by Jay Haley (*Uncommon Therapy,* W.W. Norton & Company, 1973) is recommended as a useful clarifying supplement to the content of this chapter.

Unique People Require Unique Interventions

Therapists cannot afford the lazy luxury of allowing their own needs, ideas, or preferences to determine the therapy process. The patient's potentials, knowledge, needs, and emotions are unique and therapists must have the conceptual and behavioral flexibility necessary to respect, to respond to, to utilize, or to redirect that uniqueness. Theoretical considerations, classifications, and constructs should not be allowed to define or to limit what the therapist sees or does nor should the therapist's needs or personality be allowed to do so. The therapist's personality should enter the situation only to the extent necessary to ensure that contact is made with the patient and to ensure that the strategies or techniques eventually employed by the therapist are genuine expressions of informed concern and not mere rote imitation or mechanical reproduction.

The therapist also must be dedicated enough to the welfare

of the patient to spend whatever time or energy is necessary to devise an appropriate strategy for each patient. Erickson did not rely upon short cuts or pat answers, which may be why his interventions were so effective. He often spent hours devising the specific wording he would use with a patient or considering the behavioral assignments he would give. His interventions did not spring magically from thin air but were usually the products of long periods of problem solving.

I think that true psychotherapy is knowing that each patient is an individual, unique and different.
(Zeig, 1980, p. 226)

You're going to find a tremendous divergence in your patients. Why not? People are different, understandings are different.
(ASCH, 1980, Taped Lecture, 7/16/65)

Each patient's problem needs individual scrutiny and the structuring of the therapeutic approach to meet the individuality of the problem. [1966]
(In Erickson, 1980, Vol. IV, chap. 18, p. 192)

I think that psychotherapy is an individual procedure.
(Zeig, 1980, p. 104)

You individualize your therapy to meet the needs of the individual patient.
(Zeig, 1980, p. 113)

In every psychiatric case, you have to take the individual personality into consideration.
(Erickson, 1977b, p. 32)

Any therapy used should always be in accordance with the needs of the patient, whatever they may be, and not based in any way upon arbitrary classifications. [1958]

(In Erickson, 1980, Vol. IV, chap. 15, p. 174)

But the important thing is: Deal with your patient and don't substitute your ideas.

(Zeig, 1980, p. 130)

I think that in hypnotherapy and in experimental work with subjects, you have no right to express a preference; that it is a cooperative venture of some sort, and that the personality of the subject or the patient is the thing of primary importance.

(Erickson, 1977a, p. 14)

I think the textbooks on therapy try to impress upon you a great number of concepts. Concepts that you should take from your patients, not from books, because books teach you you should do things in a certain way.

(Zeig, 1980, p. 226)

This matter of concepts of advanced psychotherapy should include this; That you ought to rely upon the capacity of the individual patient to furnish you the cues, the information by which to organize your psychotherapy because the patient can find a way if you give him an opportunity.

(ASCH, 1980, Taped Lecture, 8/14/66)

One should look upon his adult patient or his childish patient as possessing understandings that are available if you are willing to respect that patient and willing to give that patient the opportunity to make use of his capacities to function and to react to the therapeutic situation.

(ASCH, 1980, Taped Lecture, 8/14/66)

Nor does he [Erickson] know of anybody who has ever really understood the variety and purposes of any one patient's multiple symptoms despite the tendency of many psychiatrists to hypothecate, to their own satisfaction, towering structures of explanation often as elaborate and bizarre as the patient's symptomatology. [1966]

(In Erickson, 1980, Vol. IV, chap. 18, p. 202)

No person can really understand the individual patterns of learning and response of another. [1952]

(In Erickson, 1980, Vol. I, chap. 6, p. 154)

In psychotherapy, you ought to know that your patient knows more about his past learnings than you can ever know.

(Zeig, 1980, p. 46)

The ego, as far as I know, is a helpful and convenient concept, but that is all that it is. [1962]

(In Erickson, 1980, Vol. II, chap. 33, p. 340)

Now too much has been written and said and done about the re-education of the neurotic and the psychotic and the maladjusted personality as if anybody could really tell any one person how to think and how to feel and how to react in any given situation. Everybody reacts differently according to his own particular patterns, his own background of personal experience. What pleases me can displease my wife.

(ASCH, 1980, Taped Lecture, 8/14/66)

Such re-education is, of course, necessarily in terms of the patient's life experiences, his understandings, memories, attitudes, and ideas; it cannot be in terms of the therapist's ideas and opinions. [1948]

(In Erickson, 1980, Vol. IV, chap. 4, p. 39)

You need those divergent understandings. There is no exactly right or absolutely wrong approach. We know too little about human nature and human personality and human potentials to ever say "this" and only "this" is right. We need to take an inquiring, a curious, an interested, a pleasingly interested attitude toward our patients, wondering just how they are going to utilize those countless billions of brain cells they all possess, most of which they'll never be called upon in life to utilize, but which, should certain circumstances arise, they may use another few million that they never expected to use.

(ASCH, 1980, Taped Lecture, 7/16/65)

Properly, it [therapy] is not a matter of advancing particular schools of thought or of attempting to substantiate interpretative psychological theories, but simply a task of appraising a patient's problem or problems in terms of the reality in which the patient lives and in the terms of the realities of the patient's continuing future as he or she may reasonably hope for it to be. [circa 1930's]

(In Erickson, 1980, Vol. IV, chap. 54, p. 482)

The leading of the patient into this more satisfying method of living and of expressing the self is a rightful goal greatly to be desired. ... The achievement of the goal while primary, is not the only consideration. Also worthy of evaluation, planning and thought by the therapist are the matters of time spent, of effective utilization of effort, and above all of the fullest possible utilization of the functional capacities and abilities and the experiential and acquisitional learnings of the patient. These should take precedence over the teachings of new ways of living which are developed from the therapist's possibly incomplete understanding of what may be right and serviceable to the individual concerned. [1965]

(In Erickson, 1980, Vol. I, chap. 29, p. 540)

The importance in therapy of doing what appears to be most important to the patient, that which constitutes an expression of the distorted thoughts and emotions of the patient. The therapist's task should not be a proselytizing of the patient with his own beliefs and understandings. No patient can really understand the understandings of his therapist nor does he need them. What is needed is the development of a therapeutic situation permitting the patient to use his own thinking, his own understandings, his own emotions in the way that best fits him in his scheme of life. [1965]

(In Erickson, 1980, Vol. IV, chap. 20, p. 223)

She is using some material I offered, and what she uses is a function of her personality, not mine.

(Erickson & Rossi, 1979, p. 416)

Yes, I'm emphasizing her own natural memory patterns — rather than having her rely on some way of remembering she was artificially taught.

(Erickson & Rossi, 1979, p. 283)

I think she will probably put into practice the teaching she has had throughout her lifetime.

(Zeig, 1980, p. 246)

She is right about the fact that she should not let me get in the way of her using herself.

(Erickson & Rossi, 1979, p. 212)

I emphasize a patient's own functioning and feelings as a unique personality. With a series of suggestions like this you can focus the patient's attention more and more onto their own inner experiences. [1976-1978]

(In Erickson, 1980, Vol. I, chap. 23, p. 479)

I don't know the kind of thinking you ought to do.
But I think you ought to enjoy doing your own thinking
in terms of your own field of competence.

(ASCH, 1980, Taped Lecture, 7/18/65)

In any psychotherapeutic situation, whatever the
school of thought which predominated, there must be
recognized over and above the formalized structure of
thinking, the importance of the patient himself as a sen-
tient being with needs, capabilities, experiences, and a
separateness as an individual, with his own background
of experiential and acquisitional learning. He is not properly to be squeezed into any ritualistic traditional
method of procedure, nor limited by teachings governed
by predetermined rules and formulae. [1965]

(In Erickson, 1980, Vol. I, chap. 29, pp. 541–542)

And I do wish that Rogerian therapists, Gestalt
therapists, transactional analysts, group analysts, and all
the other offspring of various theories would recognize
that not one of them really recognizes that psychotherapy
for person #1 is not psychotherapy for person #2.

(Zeig, 1980, p. 104)

And all the rules of Gestalt therapy, psychoanalysis
and transactional analysis, ...many theorists write them
down in books as if every person was like every other
person.

(Zeig, 1980, p. 220)

Be willing to avoid following any *one* teaching or any
one technique.

(Haley, 1976, p. 535)

It [Hypnotic Corrective Emotional Experience] is, as is
illustrated in the instances cited, best "played by ear"

with no elaborate plans formulated, but with a multitude of possibilities floating freely in one's mind ready for adaptation to each new development presented by the patient. [1965]

(In Erickson, 1980, Vol. IV, chap. 58, p. 524)

I've treated many conditions, and I always invent a new treatment in accord with the individual personality. I know that when I take guests out to dinner, I let the guest choose what to eat, because I don't *know* what they like. I think people should dress the way they *want* to.

(Zieg, 1980, p. 104)

The variability of subjects, the individuality of their general and immediate needs, their differences in time and situation requirements, the uniqueness of their personalities and capabilities, together with the demands made by the projected work, render impossible any absolutely rigid procedure. [1952]

(In Erickson, 1980, Vol. I, chap. 6, p. 144)

Hence, to a significant degree, psychotherapy must necessarily be experimental in character since there can be no foreknowledge of the procedures exactly applicable to any one patient.

(Erickson, 1954c, p. 261)

I know that in the situation of dealing with patients I often wish I knew exactly what I was doing and why, instead of feeling, as I know I did with both patients that I was acting blindly and intuitively to elicit an as yet undetermined response with which, whatever it was, I would deal. [1966]

(In Erickson, 1980, Vol. II, chap. 34, p. 353)

One must modify his own behavior; that is, the therapist actually must be fairly fluid in his behavior, because if he is rigid he is going to elicit certain types of rigid behavior in his patient. In turn, his patient's rigid behavior is unfamiliar to him, and he is not going to be able to handle him properly. Therefore, the more fluidity in the hypnotherapist, the more easily you can actually approach the patient.

(Erickson, 1977b, p. 22)

He [the patient] wants to know if you have the right kind of strength and that means a fight. Are you meek and mild as you should be, or are you strong and combative as you should be?

(Zeig, 1980, p. 342)

You accept that prestige and enhance it indirectly because he needs it. You keep it by being very modest about it.

(Erickson & Rossi, 1981, p. 229)

A therapist should have flexibility in his schedule to accommodate the patient's needs.

(Erickson & Rossi, 1979, p. 382)

Then to meet the child's emotional needs further, I proceeded to talk to her, telling interesting things, boring things, exciting things, mildly offensive things, ridiculous things, highly intriguing things.

(Erickson & Rossi, 1979, p. 271)

Much speculative thought was given to the content of her limited understandings to devise some kind of therapeutic approach. [1965]

(In Erickson, 1980, Vol. IV, chap. 20, p. 220)

Three days of intensive thinking of what to do with an obviously brain-damaged patient...[1963]
(In Erickson, 1980, Vol. IV, chap. 30, p. 288)

Use Whatever the Patient Presents

Erickson referred to his therapeutic style as a naturalistic or utilization approach. The basic principle of his utilization approach is to *use whatever dominant beliefs, values, attitudes, emotions or behaviors the patient presents in order to develop an experience that will initiate or facilitate therapeutic change.* Although some contemporaries referred to his style as intuitive or magical, he emphasized that his approach is based upon a simple recognition of conditions as they are and a utilization of those conditions to accomplish the desired ends. Whatever the patient wants, does, or is must by accepted and utilized, according to Erickson. He offered patients what was compatible with their interests, their personalities, their understandings, and their desires and his patients responded to these offerings in the only way that they could, by accepting them and reacting to them in ways that would initiate therapeutic change.

Erickson welcomed anything the patient did or said because he viewed the patient's responses as a gift. Patients give therapists the solution to their situation if only therapists are observant enough to notice, open enough to accept, and flexible enough to utilize what the patient offers. What the patient is and what the patient does are markers indicating the easiest and perhaps the only route to therapeutic change. From Erickson's perspective, all paths do lead to Rome. The only trick is to figure out how to get to Rome on the path the patient presents.

Initially, this requires the adoption of the patient's perspective or frame of reference. When the goal of therapy is viewed from that perspective the roadblocks and open pathways may become more obvious. When the therapist operates from within the patient's perspective, the patient both feels understood and understands the therapist. In addition, when the therapist views the patient from that perspective, what the patient is willing and able to do will become more obvious and the language and behaviors necessary to move the patient in that direction will also become more apparent.

> **And you pick whatever lock is presented to you. And once one lock is picked, all the other locks become vulnerable.**
>
> *(Rossi, 1973, p. 16)*

> **In therapeutic approaches, one must always take into consideration the actual personality of the individual. One must give thought to how they express their behavior.**
> **Are they over-friendly, hostile, defiant, extroverted, introverted, so on?**
>
> *(Erickson, 1977b, p. 22)*

> **The purpose of psychotherapy should be the helping of the patient in that fashion most adequate, available and acceptable. In rendering the patient aid, there should be full respect for and utilization of whatever the patient presents.**
>
> *(Erickson, 1954d, p. 127)*

> *My learning over the years was that I tried to direct the patient too much. It took a long time to let things develop and make use of things as they developed.*
>
> *(Erickson, Rossi & Rossi, p. 265)*

The purpose and procedures of psychotherapy should involve the acceptance of what the patient represents and presents. These should be utilized to give the patient impetus and momentum so as to make his present and future become absorbing, constructive and satisfying.

(Erickson, 1954d, pp. 127–128)

You ought to start simply and let patients elaborate in accord with their own personality needs — not in accord with your concepts of what is useful to them.

(Erickson & Rossi, 1981, p. 12)

Both experimental and clinical subjects often have definite preferences which should be respected. [1964]

(In Erickson, 1980, Vol. I, chap. 10, p. 283)

In brief, whatever the behavior manifested by the subjects, it should be accepted and regarded as grist for the mill. [1952]

(In Erickson, 1980, Vol. I, chap. 6, p. 158)

Whatever the patient presents to you in the office, you really ought to use.

(Erickson & Rossi, 1981, p. 16)

One always tries to use whatever the patient brings into the office. If they bring in resistance, be grateful for that resistance. Heap it up in whatever fashion they want you to — really pile it up.

(Erickson & Rossi, 1981, p. 16)

In other words, you try to accept the patient's ideas no matter what they are, and then you can try to direct (sic — we now prefer *utilize*) them.

(Erickson & Rossi, 1981, p. 13)

If it is their way of functioning, you'd better go along with it.

(Erickson, Rossi & Rossi, 1976, p. 263)

If he wanted that type of behavior, let him have it. But I really ought to be willing to use it.

(Erickson & Rossi, 1981, p. 17)

Therapists wishing to help their patients should never scorn, condemn or reject any part of a patient's conduct because it is obstructive, unreasonable, or even irrational. The patient's behavior is a part of the problem brought into the office; it constitutes the personal environment within which therapy must take effect; it may constitute the dominant force in the total doctor-patient relationship. Since whatever patients bring into the office is in some way both a part of them and a part of their problem, the patient should be viewed with a sympathetic eye appraising the totality which confronts the therapist. [1965]

(In Erickson, 1980, Vol. IV, chap. 20, p. 213)

By naturalistic approach is meant the acceptance and utilization of the situation encountered without endeavoring to psychologically restructure it. In so doing, the presenting behavior of the patient becomes a definite aid and an actual part in inducing a trance, rather than a possible hindrance. [1958]

(In Erickson, 1980, Vol. I, chap. 7, p. 168)

There is an imperative need to accept and to utilize those psychological states, understandings and attitudes that the patient brings into the situation. ...The acceptance and utilization of those factors ... promotes more rapid trance induction, the development of more profound trance states, the more ready acceptance of therapy, and greater ease for the handling of the total therapeutic situation. [1958]

(In Erickson, 1980, Vol. I, chap. 7, p. 175-176)

My mental set in approaching the task was that of discovering what I could understand of the patient's behavior and what I could do about it or with it. [1966]

(In Erickson, 1980, Vol. II, chap. 34, p. 351)

By using the patient's own patterns of response and behavior, including those of their actual illness, one may effect therapy more promptly and satisfactorily, with resistance to therapy greatly obviated and acceptance of therapy facilitated. [1973]

(In Erickson, 1980, Vol. IV, chap. 38, p. 348)

All that I hope to know in most such experimental situations that I devise is the possible general variety of psychological processes and reactions I would like to elicit but do not know if I shall succeed in so doing, nor in what manner this will occur. Then, as the subjects respond in their own fashion, I promptly utilize that response. [1964]

(In Erickson, 1980, Vol. I, chap. 15, p. 347)

Such recognition and concession to the needs of the subjects and the utilization of their behavior do not constitute, as some authors have declared, "unorthodox techniques," based upon "clinical intuition," instead they constitute a simple recognition of existing conditions, based upon full respect for subjects as functioning personalities. [1952]

(In Erickson, 1980, Vol. I, chap. 6, p. 155)

Sometimes — in fact, many more times than is realized — therapy can be firmly established on a sound basis only by the utilization of silly, absurd, irrational, and contradictory manifestations. One's professional dignity is not involved, but one's professional competence is. [1965]

(In Erickson, 1980, Vol. IV, chap. 20, p. 213)

Yes, therapy should always be designed to fit the patient and not the patient to fit the therapy.

(Erickson & Rossi, 1979, p. 415)

I don't argue, I take their frame of reference — in the direction I want it to go. You let your subjects see everything.

(Erickson & Rossi, 1981, p. 251)

Any 52 year-old woman that starts calling me "sonny" has a sense of humor. So I made use of that.

In other words, whatever your patient has, make use of it.

(Zeig, 1980, p. 189)

When you have an intellectual subject, you stick to the intellectual. That is what he will understand and will accept. You have to fit your technique to the patient's frame of reference.

(Erickson & Rossi, 1981, p. 254)

Use the Patient's Desires and Expectations

The desires, wishes, and expectations of a patient can play at least three vital roles in the process of psychotherapy: they can provide permission for the therapist to do something about the problem, they can provide a source of motivation which the therapist can help the patient use to deal with the problem, and they can describe how the therapist should respond to the patient. The desire or need to have something done to alleviate a problem and the expectation that the therapist will do something about it usually are what brings the patient to the therapist's office in the first place. As such, they are sources of motivation that can be used to initiate other responses and they are expressions of the patient's willingness to allow the therapist to help.

However, the patient's desires and expectations often include a specification of how the patient wants or expects to be aided. It seems almost self-evident that if a patient indicates the need or expectation to have therapy conducted in a particular manner then the therapist should conduct therapy in that manner. If a patient expects the therapist to use specific techniques or to behave in particular ways, then that patient probably will be more likely to cooperate and to change if the therapist does so. In this manner the therapist uses the patient's desires and expectations to create an atmosphere and a therapeutic style tailored to that particular patient and in so doing creates a situation that has the greatest likelihood of being maximally effective.

> **These physically traumatic aspects of the experiences gave rise to an intense wish that these things would not and could not be so, that things would change completely. In response to this great need there developed the psychological processes by which, step by step, there could be utilization of repressions, overemphasis of various elements of the experience and distortion of others, until finally there had been achieved a complete reconstruction of the entire experience in a form which**

could meet the compelling needs of the personality. [1938]

> *(In Erickson, 1980, Vol. III, chap. 22, p. 227)*

Effective therapy was based upon the utilization of the personality's need for something to be done in direct relationship to the injury. [1959]

> *(In Erickson, 1980, Vol. I, chap. 8, p. 195)*

She has a very strong desire to do good work. She is strong there, so I'm using that motivation to deal with the place where she is weak — her airplane phobia.

> *(Erickson & Rossi, 1979, p. 333)*

This extremely authoritarian approach was deemed appropriate because it utilized the patient's previous life experience and current expectation that effective guidance always came in an authoritarian form.

> *(Erickson & Rossi, 1979, p. 244)*

These three different case histories are presented to illustrate the importance in therapy of doing what appears to be most important to the patient, that which constitutes an expression of the distorted thoughts and emotions of the patient. [1965]

> *(In Erickson, 1980, Vol. IV, chap. 20, p. 223)*

Use the Patient's Language

All patients have their own unique language and nonverbal behaviors. More often than not, therapists challenge and attempt to revise the language used by patients to discuss therapeutic issues. Analytic patients begin to talk like their analysts, Jungian patients adopt the Jungian vocabulary, and patients of behaviorists discuss their problems in learning-theory terms. As described earlier, however, Erickson revised this process. Rather than altering the patient's language system to suit his style, he altered his own language and behavior patterns to suit the patient's style. He actually used the same words and phrases his patients had used when he presented his thoughts and interventions to those patients.

Aside from the comforting experience of being understood and accepted that this created in his patients, his ability to use the patient's language style enabled him to communicate more effectively with patients about their problems in symbolic or metaphorical terms. If a patient used particular terms to describe a presenting problem or a therapeutic goal, Erickson would use those same terms within the context of metaphors or allegories to provide a new perspective on the problem or on the solution to that problem, sometimes without the patient's direct awareness. The personal impact of a metaphor can be much more intense and its point better understood when couched in personally relevant terms. At the same time, if the patient is not yet ready for such an understanding, the point of the metaphor, because it is not stated directly, may be overlooked for the moment but not dismissed as entirely or permanently as it could have been without the personally meaningful terms. Eventually the therapeutic significance will probably creep through.

Whether presenting metaphors or simple direct statements, Erickson ensured a high level of comprehension and impact by using the linguistic and behavioral style of each patient. Even a simple conversation is easier if both people speak the same language and in the therapeutic setting the patient's language style should be the style of choice.

Transform their own utterances into vitally important suggestions effectively guiding their behavior, although

without such recognition by them at the time. [1964]
(In Erickson, Vol. I, chap. 13, p. 300)

You are using his own words to alter the patient's access to his various frames of reference.
(Erickson & Rossi, 1981, p. 255)

The patient had told his story, and note had been taken of the patterning of his behavior as was revealed by that story. Then came the problem of devising a therapeutic procedure employing symbolic language expressive of his story. [1973]
(In Erickson, 1980, Vol. IV, chap. 38, p. 349)

It [repeating the patient's utterances] serves to comfort them with a conviction that they are secure, that nothing is being done to them or being imposed upon them, and they feel that they can comfortably be aware of every step of the procedure. Consequently they are able to give full cooperation, which would be difficult to secure if they were to feel that a pattern of behavior was being forcibly imposed upon them [1959]
(In Erickson, 1980, Vol. I, chap. 8, p. 183)

This acceptance of a patient's declaration and turning it back upon him in the form of posthypnotic suggestions is often a most effective therapeutic procedure. It gives the patient a feeling of being committed to his own intentions and wishes, and intensifies his ability to act accordingly, without a feeling that he is being forced to accept proferred help. [1954]
(In Erickson, 1980, Vol. IV, chap. 23, p. 234)

Use the Patient's Emotions

The typical emotional tendencies or actual expressions of emotion that a patient brings into the office should be considered to be a valuable potential source of motivation. The elicitation of such typical emotions will initiate behavior that, with some planning, can be directed toward therapeutic goals. Many of Erickson's patients were stirred into effective action by their angers, fears, or frustrations. If patients are willing to overcome their problems to spite their therapists but not to please them, then therapists should be willing to stimulate their spite and indignation. If other patients are motivated by guilt, then therapists should consider using that quality to motivate the desired change in thought or behavior. Therapists must work with what they have, and if what they have is an angry person, they must use that person's anger effectively. The same holds true no matter what emotion is available as a motivator.

Again, there are no secret formulae that show therapists how to use patients' emotions to motivate therapeutic change; therapists must develop this skill by doing it. Trying to stimulate the motivating emotions or interests of others and re-directing those motivations into particular actions can be a fascinating and productive daily game. Most therapists want to do more than wait for patients to decide to change or rationally debate the need for change with them. Utilization of existing motivators can provide a useful alternative.

Underlying the entire procedure was the utilization of the patient's emotions. Each new measure in some manner elicited emotional reactions, attitudes and states — sometimes pleasant, but more often of special personal

displeasure — and these were employed to intensify and promote her learnings and to stimulate her to greater effort. [1964]

(In Erickson, 1980, Vol. IV, chap. 31, p. 312

Then one should bear in mind that these patients are highly motivated, that their disinterest, antagonism, belligerence, and disbelief are actually allies in bringing about the eventual results, nor does this author ever hesitate to utilize what is offered. [1964]

(In Erickson, 1980, Vol. I, Chap. 10, p. 286

I just stirred up *his* anger and let him realize — gently — that I stirred up his anger and was stimulating him into activity. And as soon as he really understood that and really saw what he could do, his anger evaporated.

(ASCH, 1980, Taped Lecture, 7/16/65)

Anne's aggression was instantly transformed into a totally different kind of thing that offered not an opportunity for aggressive retaliative attack but a joyous participation by all others in the transformation of the aggression. Yet, Anne was, in essence, left unscathed as a person, since there still remained with her the control of the aggression.

(Erickson & Rossi, 1979, p. 360)

Her repressed and guilty resentments and hostilities toward her son and his misbehavior were utilized. Every effort was made to redirect them into an anticipation of a satisfying, calculated, deliberate watchfulness in the frustrating of her son's attempts to confirm his sense of insecurity and to prove her ineffectual. [1962]

(In Erickson, 1980, vol. IV, chap. 57, p. 511)

The rationale of the author's decision was that the patient had a well-developed pattern of frustration and despair which, properly employed, could be used constructively as a motivational force in eliciting responses with a strong and probably compelling emotional force and tone leading to actual new learnings of self-expression. [1963]

(In Erickson, 1980, Vol. IV, chap. 30, p. 289)

Capitalizing upon her frustration and despair by employing measures which might conceivably make use of resulting strong emotional drives as a basis of evoking a great variety of response patterns and of motivating learning. [1963]

(In Erickson, 1980, Vol. IV, chap. 30, p. 311)

Frustration was used deliberately to prevent despair by compelling the patient, in self-protection, to strive to secure some satisfaction of ordinary, reasonable and legitimate desires. [1963]

(In Erickson, 1980, Vol. IV, chap. 30, p. 309)

This type of cavalier offer to help him utilized his need for inferiority even in the therapeutic situation and actually pleased him. [1937–38]

(In Erickson, 1980, Vol. IV, chap. 55, p. 492)

Use the Patient's Resistance

One of Erickson's most noteworthy attributes as a professional was his ability to work effectively with highly resistant patients. Most therapists are completely frustrated by a total lack of cooperation, but Erickson accepted resistance and utilized it to effect therapeutic progress. He had no magical powers for doing this; he simply acknowledged the patient's right to resist and then arranged circumstances in such a manner that in order to resist, patients had to respond in a therapeutically beneficial way. He permitted their resistance, even encouraged it, because he knew he could redirect it to suit the patient's therapeutic needs.

> **Since negativity was the dominant mental set, it was the most effective one to achieve the desired results.**
>
> *(Erickson & Rossi, 1979, p. 363)*

> **Such resistance should be openly accepted, in fact, graciously accepted, since it is a vitally important communication of a part of their problems and often can be used as an opening into their defenses. This is something that the patients do not realize. [1964]**
>
> *(In Erickson, 1980, Vol. I, chap. 13, p. 299)*

> **Resistances constituting a part of the problem can be utilized by enhancing them and thereby permitting the patient to discover, under guidance, new ways of behavior favorable to recovery. [1948]**
>
> *(In Erickson, 1980, Vol. IV, chap. 4, p. 48)*

> **The therapist who is aware of this, particularly if well skilled in hypnotherapy, can easily and often quickly transform these overt, seemingly uncooperative forms of behavior into a good rapport, a feeling of being understood, and an attitude of hopeful expectancy of successfully achieving the goals being sought. [1964]**
>
> *(In Erickson, 1980, Vol. I, chap. 13, p. 299)*

> **His hostile manner and attitude suggested the inadvisability of attempting any routine traditional technique. [1936]**
>
> *(In Erickson, 1980, Vol. IV, chap. 26, p. 253)*

> Why shouldn't I give her something to reject? I think whenever you have a patient who is rejecting, who is antagonistic, who is resisting, you ought to appreciate the fact that they are antagonistic. And you ought to be able to mention antagonism and resentment in such a fashion that they can take the initiative in rejecting that antagonism, in rejecting that resistance and in achieving the relaxation that you want them to achieve.
>
> *(ASCH, 1980, Taped Lecture, 2/2/66)*

Use the Patient's Symptoms

Like all other aspects of patients' response styles, their symptomatology can be therapeutic ammunition. Symptoms often can be used to initiate therapeutic change or can be transformed into useful or more manageable responses. Anxieties, phobias, delusions, and all other symptoms constitute important and compelling features of the individual's experiential life. Rather than attacking them or overlooking them, the therapist may be able to utilize them therapeutically. The psychological, emotional, and behavioral energy underlying these symptoms can become a beneficial source of impetus for change if used creatively. Even pathological symptoms must be accepted at times as a necessary feature of that particular individual's personality. Rather than expending the inordinate amount of time and energy it might take to reorganize the person's personality to the extent necessary to eliminate the sympton, it may be wise to transform the expression of the underlying pathology into less disruptive behaviors. For example, replacing an hysterical paralysis of the right arm with an hysterical paralysis of the third joint of the left little finger may be a satisfactory solution for everyone involved. Hating the therapist may be a satisfactory alternative to hating everybody. Transformation of a pathological thought, emotion or behavior into an insignificant manifestation often is the most pragmatic solution.

A short summary of Erickson's attitude is that *anything that occurs in the therapy session can be used to initiate therapeutic movement,* be it resistance, anger, a preferred topic of conversation, a behavior, or even an error on the part of the therapist. No matter what happens, therapists should be ready to twist it in a direction that will turn it into a therapeutic occurrence.

> **This author has repeatedly stressed the importance of utilizing patients' symptoms and general patterns of behavior in psychotherapy. Such utilization renders unnecessary any effort to alter or transform symptomatology as a preliminary measure to the reeducation of patients in relation to the crucial problems confronting them in their illness. Such problems cause a distortion of their thinking, feeling, and patterns of living, thereby causing them to seek therapy. [1973]**
>
> *(In Erickson, 1980, Vol. IV, chap. 38, p. 348)*

> **Therapy had to be based upon an apparently complete acceptance of the symptoms, and it was achieved by ameliorating the symptoms.**
>
> *(Erickson, 1954d, p. 117)*

> **Consequently, the therapeutic task becomes a problem of intentionally utilizing neurotic symptomatology to meet the unique needs of the patient. Such utilization must satisfy the compelling desire for neurotic handicaps, the limitations imposed upon therapy by external forces, and, above all, provide adequately for constructive adjustments aided rather than handicapped by the continuance of neuroticisms.**
>
> *(Erickson, 1954d, p. 109)*

There is a utilization of neurotic behavior by a transformation of the personality purposes it serves without an attack upon the symptomatology itself.

(Erickson, 1954d, p. 112)

Therefore, as therapy, there was substituted for the existing neurotic disability another, comparable in kind, nonincapacitating in character, and symptomatically satisfying to them as constructively functioning personalities.

(Erickson, 1954d, p. 112)

Utilizing the patient's own neurotic irrationality to affirm and confirm a simple extension of his neurotic fixation relieved him of all unrecognized unconscious needs to defend his neuroticism against all assaults. [1965]

(In Erickson, 1980, Vol. IV, chap. 20, p. 218)

For both patients, the utilization of anxiety by a continuance and a transformation of it provided for a therapeutic resolution into a normal emotion permitting a normal adjustment.

(Erickson, 1954d, p. 116)

Therapy was accomplished by systematically utilizing this anxiety through a process of redirecting and transforming it.

(Erickson, 1954d, p. 116)

One tries to make it possible for the patient to exercise his own ambivalence for your benefit and for his benefit.

(Erickson & Rossi, 1981, p. 4)

Use Your Own Observations

Therapists should enter the therapy situation with a backlog of observations about people. There are some general patterns of stimuli and response that will hold true across populations and that thus will apply to each patient. This knowledge should be used by the therapist whenever possible to elicit generally predictable responses that will promote or represent therapeutic change for that particular patient.

Therapists must observe each patient carefully but they must also observe carefully the everyday behavior of people in order to discover the common reactions to various situations, events, and words. This generalized knowledge can be used later to initiate desired therapeutic responses or to guide the patient's attention and experience in the necessary directions. Erickson's observations about people in Section I can serve as a starting point for the further accumulation of useful observations by each therapist. Much of the data in the psychological research literature can serve a similar purpose. Ultimately, however, therapists must assume personal responsibility for observing carefully and accumulating general information that will be meaningful and useful to them. Similar observations, of course, must be made rapidly and efficiently about each patient.

Stimulating therapeutic change in an Ericksonian manner actually involves the application of rather mechanical skills. They are admittedly complex skills requiring an extensive background of observation and experience, but all therapy really amounts to is pushing the perceptual, emotional, intellectual, and behavioral buttons that the therapist is already reasonably sure will cause the desired therapeutic reactions and experiential learnings on the part of the patient. The therapist simply becomes so familiar with the general operation of people and with the peculiar motivations and response patterns of each patient that by word and deed, the therapist can push the buttons that experience and observation have taught will generate the needed reactions.

> **In every attempt at psychotherapy there is always the need to utilize the common experiences and understandings that permeate the pattern of daily living, and to adapt such utilization to the unique needs of the individual patient.**
>
> *(Erickson, 1954c, p. 261)*

> **Suggesting eight hours of rest also utilizes what we experience in everyday life. You frequently sleep on something in order to deal with it.**
>
> *(Erickson & Rossi, 1979, p. 325)*

> **Now, there is nothing magical about what I did — *it was a recognition of the thinking Cathy would do...* the thinking and the understanding that would derive out of Cathy's ordinary life. A woman who grew up in this culture, in this age, would have certain learnings as a result of just being alive.**
>
> *(Erickson & Rossi, 1979, p. 137)*

Summary

The problem confronting therapists is how to say or to do something that will initiate an experience from which the patient can benefit. The goal may be to confront patients with their unused or misused capacities, to force them into a reevaluation of their beliefs or assumptions or to alter their inappropriate behaviors but, no matter what aspect of reality requires a more objective appraisal or response, it remains the therapist's job to provide an experience that will move patients in a behavioral, emotional, or intellectual direction they have been unable or unwilling to move in previously.

Erickson's solution to this problem consisted entirely of his willingness to accept and to utilize whatever responses were typical or normal for the patient. He tried to use whatever attitudes, interests, emotions, or symptoms the patient brought into his office. If anger was the patient's predominant characteristic, he used that anger. If the patient's pride was noticeable, he used that. If his patients were interested in gardening or travel, he used that. He even adopted and used the language style of his patients. He allowed his patients to determine the dominant characteristics of the therapeutic context and then used those characteristics to initiate or trigger a therapeutic experience.

The creativity involved in transforming or redirecting whatever the patient presents into a therapeutic response should not be underestimated. In fact, the conceptual problem involved is the same type of problem frequently encountered in tests of creativity, i.e., "Given these tools, how do you accomplish that task?" Careful observation to notice the primary motives, needs, attitudes, etc. of other people and considerable conceptual flexibility to adopt their perspectives and language patterns are also necessary. Therapeutic intervention requires a combination of all these abilities: creativity, observation, and flexibility as well as practice and a willingness to take risks.

Effective teachers seem to be especially adept at presenting information within a context that has some personal significance or importance to their students. They allow their students to experience things that demonstrate the truth of what they are saying in a direct and undeniable fashion. Good teachers can make any topic personally relevant and can package any material in an appealing and motivating manner. The parallels seem obvious and may account for Erickson's tendency to focus upon the therapist's role as teacher. His patients learned things that were therapeutic; they were not "cured" by him. He always spoke of the therapy process as a learning process. Perhaps as we begin to think of ourselves as teachers, the utilization technique and the general set of attitudes underlying it will become more comprehensible and usable.

REFERENCES

American Society of Clinical Hypnosis (Producer) *Milton H. Erickson classic cassette series*. 1980, Audio taped lectures by Dr. Erickson from 8/8/64, 7/16/65, 7/18/65, 2/2/66 and 8/14/66.

Bandler, R. & Grinder, J. *Patterns of the hypnotic techniques of Milton H. Erickson, M.D.,* Cupertine, Cal.: Meta Publications, 1975.

Beahrs, J.O. Integrating Erickson's approach. *American Journal of Clinical Hypnosis*, 1977, *20,* 55–68.

Erickson, M.H. A brief survey of hypnotism. *Medical Record,* 1934, *140,* 609–613.

Erickson, M.H. An experimental investigation of the possible anti-social use of hypnosis. *Psychiatry*, 1939a, *2,* 391–414.

Erickson, M.H. The application of hypnosis to psychiatry. *Medical Record*, 1939b, *150,* 60–65.

Erickson, M.H. The early recognition of mental disease. *Diseases of the Nervous System*, 1941a, *2,* 99–108.

Erickson, M.H. Hypnosis: a general review. *Diseases of the Nervous System*, 1941b, *2,* 13–18.

Erickson, M.H. The therapy of a psychosomatic headache. *Journal of Clinical and Experimental Hypnosis*, 1953, *4,* 2–6.

Erickson, M.H. A clinical note on indirect hypnotic therapy. *Journal of Clinical and Experimental Hypnosis*, 1954a, *2,* 171–174.

Erickson, M.H. Hypnotism. Encyclopaedia Britannica, 14th edition, Vol. 12, 1954b, 22–24.

Erickson, M.H. Pseudo-orientation in time as on hypnotherapeutic procedure. *Journal of Clinical and Experimental Hypnosis*, 1954c, *2,* 261–283.

Erickson, M.H. Special techniques of brief hypnotherapy. *Journal of Clinical and Experimental Hypnosis*, 1954d, *2*, 109-129.

Erickson, M.H. Self-exploration in the hypnotic state. *Journal of Clinical and Experimental Hypnosis*, 1955, *3*, 49-57.

Erickson, M.H. Hypnosis. *Encyclopaedia Britannica,* 14th Edition, Vol. 11, 1970, 995-997 (also in 14th Edition, 1961, Vol. 12, 23-24A).

Erickson, M.H. A field investigation by hypnosis of sound loci importance in human behavior. *American Journal of Clinical Hypnosis*, 1973, *16*, 92-109.

Erickson, M.H. Control of physiological functions by hypnosis. *American Journal of Clinical Hypnosis*. 1977a, *20*, 8-19.

Erickson, M.H. Hypnotic approaches to therapy. *American Journal of Clinical Hypnosis*. 1977b, *20*, 20-35.

Erickson, M.H. *The collected papers of Milton H. Erickson on hypnosis* (4 vols.) (Edited by Ernest L. Rossi). New York: Irvington Publishers, 1980.

(Listed below by volume and chapter are the original references for all of Dr. Erickson's articles reprinted in this four-volume collection from which quotations were obtained for the present book.)

VOLUME I

Chapters

1. Initial experiments investigating the nature of hypnosis. *American Journal of Clinical Hypnosis,* 1964, *7*, 152-162.

2. Further experimental investigations of hypnosis: Hypnotic and nonhypnotic realities. *American Journal of Clinical Hypnosis*, 1967, *10*, 87–135.

3. A special inquiry with Aldous Huxley into the nature and character of various states of consciousness. *American Journal of Clinical Hypnosis*, 1965, *8*, 14–33.

4. Autohypnotic experiences of Milton H. Erickson. *American Journal of Clinical Hypnosis*, 1977, *20*, 1, 36–54 (with E. L. Rossi).

5. Historical note on hand levitation and other ideomotor techniques. *American Journal of Clinical Hypnosis*, 1961, *3*, 196–199.

6. Deep hypnosis and its induction. In L.M. LeCron (Ed.) *Experimental Hypnosis*. New York: MacMillan, 1952. Pp. 70–114.

7. Naturalistic techniques of hypnosis. *American Journal of Clinical Hypnosis*, 1958, *1*, 3–8.

8. Further clinical techniques of hypnosis: Utilization techniques. *American Journal of Clinical Hypnosis*, 1959, *2*, 3–21.

9. A transcript of a trance induction with commentary. *American Journal of Clinical Hypnosis*, 1959, *2*, 49–84 (with J. Haley and J.H. Weakland).

10. The confusion technique in hypnosis. *American Journal of Clinical Hypnosis*, 1964, *6*, 183–207.

11. The dynamics of visualization, levitation and confusion in trance induction. Unpublished fragment, circa 1940's.

12. Another example of confusion in trance induction. As told to Rossi in 1976.

13. An hypnotic technique for resistant patients: The patient, the technique and its rationale, and field ex-

periments. *American Journal of Clinical Hypnosis*, 1964, *7*, 8–32.

14. Pantomime techniques in hypnosis and the implications. *American Journal of Clinical Hypnosis*, 1964, *7*, 64–70.

15. The "surprise" and "my-friend-John" techniques of hypnosis: Minimal cues and natural field experimentation. *American Journal of Clinical Hypnosis*, 1964, *6*, 293–307.

16. Respiratory rhythm in trance induction: The role of minimal sensory cues in normal and trance behavior. Unpublished fragment, circa 1960's.

17. An indirect induction of trance: Simulation and the role of indirect suggestion and minimal cues. Unpublished paper written in the 1960's.

18. Notes on minimal cues in vocal dynamics and memory. Unpublished material written in 1964.

19. Concerning the nature and character of post-hypnotic behavior. *Journal of General Psychology*, 1941, *24*, 95–133 (with E. M. Erickson).

20. Varieties of double-bind. *American Journal of Clinical Hypnosis*, 1975, *17*, 144–157 (with E. L. Rossi).

21. Two level communication and the microdynamics of trance and suggestion. *American Journal of Clinical Hypnosis*, 1976, *18*, 153–171 (with E. L. Rossi).

22. Indirect forms of suggestion. Paper presented at 28th Annual Meeting of the Society for Clinical and Experimental Hypnosis, 1976 (with E. L. Rossi).

23. Indirect forms of suggestion in hand levitation. Unpublished paper with E. L. Rossi. 1976–78.

24. Possible detrimental effects from experimental hypnosis, *Journal of Abnormal and Social Psychology*, 1932, *27*, 321–327.

VOLUME II

Chapters

ed response technique. *Journal of General Psychology*, 1938, *19*, 151–167.

12. Chemo-anesthesia in relation to hearing and memory. *American Journal of Clinical Hypnosis,* 1963, *6*, 31–36.

13. A field investigation by hypnosis of sound loci importance in human behavior. *American Journal of Clinical Hypnosis*, 1973, 16, *92–109.*

14. Hypnotic investigation of psychosomatic phenomena: Psychosomatic interrelationships studied by experimental hypnosis. *Psychosomatic Medicine*, 1943, *5*, 51–58.

18. Control of physiological functions by hypnosis. *American Journal of Clinical Hypnosis,* 1977, *20*, 1, 8–19.

19. The hypotic alteration of blood flow: An experiment comparing waking and hypnotic responsiveness. Paper presented at the American Society of Clinical Hypnosis Annual Meeting, 1958.

20. A clinical experimental approach to psychogenic infertility. Paper presented at the American Society of Clinical Hypnosis Annual Meeting, 1958.

21. Breast development possibly influenced by hypnosis: Two instances and the psychotherapeutic results. *American Journal of Clinical Hypnosis*, 1960, *11*, 157–159.

23. The appearance in three generations of an atypical pattern of the sneezing reflex. *Journal of Genetic Psychology*, 1940, *56*, 455–459.

29. Clinical and experimental trance: Hypnotic training and time required for their development. Unpublished discussion, circa 1960.

30. Laboratory and clinical hyposis: The same or different phenomena? *American Journal of Clinical Hypnosis*, 1967, *9*, 166–170.

31. Explorations in hypnosis research. Paper presented at the Seventh Annual University of Kansas Institute for Research in Clinical Psychology in Hypnosis and Clinical Psychology, May, 1960.
32. Expectancy and minimal sensory cues in hypnosis. Incomplete report written in the 1960's.
33. Basic psychological problems in hypnotic research. In Estabrooks, G., *Hypnosis: Current Problems*. New York: Harper and Row, 1962. Pp. 207–223.
34. The experience of interviewing in the presence of observers. In L. A. Gottschalk and A. H. Aeurbach (Eds.), *Methods of Research in Psychotherapy*. New York: Appleton-Century-Crofts, 1966. Pp. 61–64.

VOLUME III

Chapters

1. A brief survey of hypnotism. *Medical Record*, 1934, 140, 609–613.
2. Hypnosis: A general review. *Diseases of the Nervous System*, 1941, *2*, 13–18.
4. The basis of hypnosis. Panel discussion on hypnosis. *Northwest Medicine*, 1959, 1404–1408.
5. The investigation of a specific amnesia. *British Journal of Medical Psychology*, 1933, *13, 143–150.*
6. Development of apparent unconsciousness during hypnotic reliving of a traumatic experience. *Archives of Neurology and Psychiatry*, 1937, *38*, 1282–1288.
7. Clinical and experimental observations on hypnotic amnesia: Introduction to an unpublished paper. Circa 1950's.

8. The problem of amnesia in waking and hypnotic states. Unpublished manuscript, circa 1960's.
9. Varieties of hypnotic amnesia. *American Journal of Clinical Hypnosis*, 1974, *16*, 225–239 (with E. L. Rossi).
10. Literalness: An experimental study. Unpublished manuscript, circa 1940's.
11. Literalness and the use of trance in neurosis. Dialogue with E. L. Rossi, 1973.
13. Past weekday determination in hypnotic and waking states. Unpublished manuscript with A. Erickson, 1962.
16. The experimental demonstration of unconscious mentation by automatic writing. *Psychoanaltyic Quarterly*, 1937, *6*, 513–529.
17. The use of automatic drawing in the interpretation and relief of a state of acute obsessional depression. *Psychoanalytic Quarterly*, 1938, *7*, 443–466 (with L. S. Kubie).
18. The translation of the automatic writing of one hypnotic subject by another in a trance-like dissociated state. *Psychoanalytic Quarterly*, 1940, *9*, 51–63 (with L. S. Kubie).
19. Experimental demonstrations of the psychopathology of everyday life. *Psychoanalytic Quarterly*, 1939, *8*, 338–353.
20. Demonstration of mental mechanisms by hypnosis. *Archives of Neurology and Psychiatry*, 1939, *42*, 367–370.
21. Unconscious mental activity in hypnosis—psychoanaltyic implications. *Psychoanalytic Quarterly*, January, 1944, Vol. XIII, No. 1 (with L. B. Hill).
22. Negation or reversal of legal testimony. *Archives of Neurology and Psychiatry*, 1938, *40*, 549–555.

23. The permanent relief of an obsessional phobia by means of communication with an unsuspected dual personality. *Psychoanalytic Quarterly*, 1939, *8*, 471–509 (with L. S. Kubie).
24. The clinical discovery of a dual personality. Unpublished manuscript, circa 1940's.
28. A study of an experimental neurosis hypnotically induced in a case of ejaculatio praecox. *British Journal of Medical Psychology*, 1935, *15*, 34–50.
29. The method employed to formulate a complex story for the induction of an experimental neurosis in a hypnotic subject. *Journal of General Psychology*, 1944, *31*, 67–84.

VOLUME IV

Chapters

1. The applications of hypnosis to psychiatry. *Medical Record,* 1939, *150*, 60–65.
2. Hypnosis in medicine. *Medical Clinics of North America.* New York: W. B. Saunders Co., 1944, 639–652.
3. Hypnotic techniques for the therapy of acute psychiatric disturbances in war. *American Journal of Psychiatry*, 1945, *101*, 668–672. (copyright 1945, American Psychiatric Association)
4. Hypnotic psychotherapy. *Medical Clinics of North America.* New York: W. B. Saunders Co., 1948, 571–584.
5. Hypnosis in general practice. *State of Mind.* 1957, 1.
6. Hypnosis: Its renascence as a treatment modality. *American Journal of Clinical Hypnosis*, 1970, *13*, 71–89. (Originally published in *Trends in Psychiatry*, Merck, Sharp & Dohme, 1966, 3 (3), 3–43.

7. Hypnotic approaches to therapy. *American Journal of Clinical Hypnosis*, 1977, *20*, 1, 20-35.

10. Experimental hypnotherapy in Tourette's Disease. *American Journal of Clinical Hypnosis*, 1965, *7*, 325-331.

11. Hypnotherapy: The patient's right to both success and failure. *American Journal of Clinical Hypnosis*, 1965, *7*, 254-257.

12. Successful hypnotherapy that failed. *American Journal of Clinical Hypnosis*, 1966, *9*, 62-65.

15. Pediatric Hypnotherapy. *American Journal of Clinical Hypnosis*, 1959, *1*, 25-29.

16. The utilization of patient behavior in the hypnotherapy of obesity: three case reports. *American Journal of Clinical Hypnosis*, 1960, *3*, 112-116.

17. Hypnosis and examination panics. *American Journal of Clinical Hypnosis*, 1965, *7*, 356-358.

18. Experiential knowledge of hypnotic phenomena employed for hypnotherapy. *American Journal of Clinical Hypnosis*, 1966, *8*, 299-309.

19. The burden of responsibility in effective psychotherapy. *American Journal of Clinical Hypnosis*, 1964, *6*, 269-271.

20. The use of symptoms as an integral part of therapy. *American Journal of Clinical Hypnosis*, 1965, *8*, 57-65.

21. Hypnosis in obstetrics: Utilizing experiential learnings. Unpublished manuscript, circa 1950's.

22. A therapeutic double bind utilizing resistance. Unpublished manuscript, 1952.

23. Utilizing the patient's own personality and ideas: "Doing it his own way." Unpublished manuscript, 1954.

24. An introduction to the study and application of hypnosis for pain control. In J. Lassner (Ed.), *Hypnosis and Psychosomatic Medicine: Proceedings of the Interna-*

tional Congress for Hypnosis and Psychosomatic Medicine. Springer Verlag, 1967.

26. Migraine headache in a resistant patient. Unpublished manuscript, 1936

27. Hypnosis in painful terminal illness. *American Journal of Clinical Hypnosis*, 1959, *1*, 117–121.

28. The interspersal hypnotic technique for symptom correction and pain control. *American Journal of Clinical Hypnosis*, 1966, *8*, 198–209.

29. Hypnotic training for transforming the experience of chronic pain. Dialogue with E. L. Rossi, 1973.

30. Hypnotically oriented psychotherapy in organic brain damage. *American Journal of Clinical Hypnosis*, 1963, *6*, 92–112.

31. Hypnotically oriented psychotherapy in organic brain damage: An addendum. *American Journal of Clinical Hypnosis*. 1964, *6*, 361–362.

33. Experimental hypnotherapy in speech problems: A case report. *American Journal of Clinical Hypnosis*, 1965, *7*, 358–360.

34. Provocation as a means of motivating recovery from a cerebrovascular accident. Unpublished manuscript, circa 1965.

35. Hypnotherapy with a psychotic. Unpublished manuscript, circa 1940's with dialogue with E. L. Rossi added later.

36. Symptom prescription for expanding the psychotic's world view. Portion of a paper with J. Zeig presented to the 20th Annual Scientific Meeting of the American Society of Clinical Hypnosis, 1977.

38. Psychotherapy achieved by a reversal of the neurotic processes in a case of ejaculatio praecox. *American Journal of Clinical Hypnosis*, 1973, *15*, 217–222.

39. Modesty: An authoritarian approach permitting recon-

ditioning via fantasy. Unpublished manuscript, circa 1950's.

40. Sterility: A therapeutic reorientation to sexual satisfaction. Unpublished manuscript, circa 1950's.

41. The abortion issue: Facilitating unconscious dynamics permitting real choice. Unpublished manuscript, circa 1950's.

42. Impotence: Facilitating unconscious reconditioning. Unpublished manuscript, 1953.

44. Vasectomy: A detailed illustration of a therapeutic reorientation. Unpublished manuscript, circa 1950's.

46. Facilitating objective thinking and new frames of reference with pseudo-orientation in time. Unpublished manuscript, circa 1940's.

49. The reorganization of unconscious thinking without awareness: Two cases with intellectualized resistance against hypnosis. Unpublished manuscript, 1956.

50. Rossi, E.L. Psychological shocks and creative moments in psychotherapy. *American Journal of Clinical Hypnosis*, 1973, *16*, 1, 9–22.

51. Facilitating a new cosmetic frame of reference. Unpublished manuscript, 1927.

52. The ugly duckling: Transforming the self-image. Unpublished manuscript, 1933.

53. A shocking breakout of a mother domination. Unpublished manuscript, circa 1936.

54. Shock and surprise facilitating a new self-image. Unpublished manuscript, circa 1930's..

55. Correcting an inferiority complex. Unpublished manuscript, 1937–1938.

56. The hypnotherapy of two psychosomatic dental problems. *Journal of the American Society of Psychosomatic Dentistry and Medicine.* 1955, *1*, 6–10.

57. The identification of a secure reality. *Family Process*, 1962, *1*, 294–303.
58. The hypnotic corrective emotional experience. *American Journal of Clinical Hypnosis*, 1965, *7*, 242–248.

Erickson, M.H. & Lustig, H.S. *Verbatim transcript of the "Artistry of Milton H. Erickson, M.D." (2 Parts)* 1975.

Erickson, M.H. & Rossi, E.L. Varieties of double bind. *American Journal of Clinical Hypnosis*, 1975, *17*, 143–157.

Erickson, M.H. & Rossi, E.L. Two level communication and the microdynamics of trance and suggestion. *American Journal of Clinical Hypnosis*, 1976, *18* 153–171.

Erickson, M.H. & Rossi, E.L. Autohypnotic experiences of Milton H. Erickson. *American Journal of Clinical Hypnosis,* 1977, *20*, 36–54.

Erickson, M.H. & Rossi, E.L. *Hypnotherapy: An Exploratory Casebook.* New York: Irvington Publishers, 1979.

Erickson, M.H. & Rossi, E.L. *Experiencing Hypnosis.* New York: Irvington Publishers, 1981.

Erickson, M.H., Rossi, E.L. & Rossi, S.I. *Hypnotic Realities.* New York: Irvington Publishers, 1976.

Haley, J. (Ed.). *Advanced Techniques of Hypnosis and Therapy.* New York: Grune & Stratton, 1967.

Rossi, E.L. Psychological shocks and creative moments in psychotherapy. *American Journal of Clinical Hypnosis,* 1973, *16*, 9-22.

Zeig, J.K. *A Teaching Seminar With Milton H. Erickson.* New York: Brunner/Mazel, 1980.

INDEX

Vigilance, 38, 41

Waking responsiveness, 40
Welfare of patients, 171-176

NOW AVAILABLE

Principles of Self Hypnosis
Pathways to the Unconscious

by C. Alexander Simpkins, Ph.D. and Annellen M. Simpkins, Ph.D.

Most self hypnosis books are incomplete. They show readers how to use their conscious mind to dominate the unconscious mind but fail to deal with the unconscious directly. In this book, the reader is shown how to experiment with the unconscious mind, unfettered by the conscious mind when appropriate. Trance is used with conscious direct suggestion, unconscious indirect suggestion, and induced free flow of associations.

The book offers an in depth history of hypnosis with special emphasis on the development of self hypnosis. Readers are also given information on the unconscious, learning, mind/body, and other topics to help them understand and creatively use self hypnosis.

Exercises throughout can be used verbatim or as guidelines for the reader's own creative associations.

An unusually lucid presentation and integration! The authors present ways to apply the techniques developed in the book to common applications and they consistently use the therapeutic trance as the primary source for learning.

Ernest L. Rossi, Ph.D., Editor of
The Collected Papers of Milton H. Erickson

ISBN 0-8290-2415-8 (Cloth)
234 pages
$19.95

AUDIO CASSETTE OFFER
Audio by C. Alexander Simpkins, Ph.D. and Annellen M. Simpkins, Ph.D.
An audio cassette, a companion to the book *Principles of Self Hypnosis*, is available, separately, for $20.00. Add another dimension to your self hypnotic instruction by listening to this tape. First your questions and concerns about self hypnosis are discussed. Then you will be imaginatively guided through suggestion and trance experiences, which are directly related to the book. Total running time, 60 minutes.

IRVINGTON PUBLISHERS, INC.
740 Broadway, New York, NY 10003

MC/Visa orders may be
telephoned to (603) 669-5933.

VOL. II

ALSO AVAILABLE

THE WISDOM OF MILTON H. ERICKSON
VOLUME 1
Hypnosis and Hypnotherapy
Edited by Ronald A. Havens

The psychiatrist Milton Erickson was a master hypnotist, capable of inducing trances by the most unexpected means—even a mere handshake. Erickson also published numerous books, articles, transcripts, and audiotapes. *The Wisdom of Milton H. Erickson I: Hypnosis and Hypnotherapy* is the first work to provide a unified survey of the philosophy behind Erickson's techniques.

The material in this volume has been selected from the psychiatrist's lectures, seminars, articles, and books and is carefully organized to offer a clear account of how Erickson conceived of hypnosis, particularly its access to the unconscious and its role in the process of psychotherapy. The reader discovers what hypnosis actually does, explores general considerations on inducing the state, learns specific techniques, and most importantly, comes to understand the contribution that hypnosis can make in the healing or therapeutic process. *The Wisdom of Milton H. Erickson I: Hypnosis and Hypnotherapy* is a valuable guide to the work of one of psychiatry's most original and innovative minds.

...a heroic effort to bring clarity to a hard-to-grasp theory...(This book) is a major reference for students and scholars who want to know what Erickson said and when and where he said it. —Contemporary Psychology

MILTON H. ERICKSON was the founder of the American Society of Clinical Hypnosis and was a life fellow of the American Psychiatric Association. He received his M.D. from the University of Wisconsin and was founding editor of the *American Journal of Clinical Hypnosis*. Erickson's books have been translated into Swedish, Italian, French, and German.

RONALD A. HAVENS is Associate Professor of Psychology at Sangamon State University and is in private practice in Springfield, Illinois. He is also the editor of *The Wisdom of Milton H. Erickson I: Hypnosis and Hypnotherapy.*

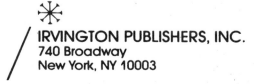

IRVINGTON PUBLISHERS, INC.
740 Broadway
New York, NY 10003

ISBN 0-8290-2413-1